A Beginner's Guide to Mindfulness

Live in the Moment

Ernst Bohlmeijer &
Monique Hulsbergen

Open University Press

Open University Press
McGraw-Hill Education
McGraw-Hill House
Shoppenhangers Road
Maidenhead
Berkshire
England
SL6 2QL

email: enquiries@openup.co.uk
world wide web: www.openup.co.uk

and Two Penn Plaza, New York, NY 10121-2289, USA

Voluit Leven, first edition by Ernst Bohlmeijer & Monique Hulsbergen

English language of *Voluit Leven* by Ernst Bohlmeijer & Monique Hulsbergen

Translation from Dutch by Sue Anderson.

A catalogue record of this book is available from the British Library

ISBN-13: 978-0-33-524735-6
ISBN-10: 0-33-524735-0
eISBN: 978-0-33-524736-3
Library of Congress Cataloging-in-Publication Data
CIP data applied for

Typesetting and e-book compilations by
RefineCatch Limited, Bungay, Suffolk
Printed by CPI Ltd

Contents

Part 2
Resources for living in the moment

Part 3
Living in the moment in practice

Foreword

As a Consultant Psychologist I work in both private practice and a large NHS hospital. My clients come from all walks of life, business executives, teachers, unemployed people, lawyers, cleaners, accountants, administrators, trades people, doctors and nurses. No one is immune from stress, anxiety and depression, which is why *A Beginner's Guide to Mindfulness: Live in the Moment* by Ernst Bohlmeijer and Monique Hulsbergen is a book that all of us can learn from.

Ernst and Monique have written a wonderful self-help guide. Full of interesting anecdotes, helpful case studies and useful techniques this book helps us to become fully acquainted with mindfulness. Divided into three sections the book takes us on a journey. Part one allows us to understand how important living in the moment is if we are to lead a satisfying life. Part two teaches us how to accept life's difficulties without becoming resigned to a negative fate. Finally, in part three we are invited to develop our own philosophy of what we want from life based upon the values that are important to us.

My late friend Richard Jones was a teacher and school counsellor. When counselling his young clients 'Jonesy', would tell the following story that described the essence of mindfulness. John, a young man in his late teens was enjoying a gap year before taking up his place at university. Whilst on his travels John had the opportunity to go white water rafting. On arriving at the river the participants including John were met by Brett an extrovert American. Brett issued everyone with helmets and life-vests before briefing them. This was to be a battle with the river Brett announced, they would have to fight hard to maintain their course as they travelled down the rapidly moving water in an attempt to avoid being smashed against the rocks by the cruel currents. They would need to respond to every instruction that Brett shouted as they fought their way to the journey's end.

John clambered into the raft and thoroughly enjoyed his experience of paddling madly against the swift running water whilst Brett yelled instructions to the crew on how to defeat the river. At the end there were high-fives and whoops of delight as the exhausted crew celebrated victory over the river.

John enjoyed his experience so much that he decided to repeat it a few days later. He was initially quite disappointed when he was greeted by Glenn a quietly spoken New Zealander with a very different approach. Glenn explained that rafting involved working with the river, allowing it to take them along – literally going with the flow. They would need to steer the raft using their paddles, the river would become their companion and they would use its energy to carry them along.

The crew set off under Glenn's quiet instructions and whilst traversing the river Glenn pointed out beautiful plants and wildlife that John had completely failed to notice the day before. At the end of the journey John was amazed how much more fulfilling his experience was under Glenn's guidance.

The river represents life's challenges – we can either engage in a battle with life or we can learn to go with the flow. The quiet voices of Ernst and Monique, with their sage advice and gentle humour, help us to understand how accepting life's challenges, rather than constantly fighting against them, allows us ultimately to lead a more contented and satisfying life.

Dr Rick Norris
Consultant Psychologist and author of
*Think Yourself Happy – The Simple 6-Stage
Programme To Change Your Life From Within*

Acknowledgments

First of all, we would like to thank the many participants in *Living in the Moment* courses in the Netherlands who test-drove the first version of this book and took time to respond and comment. This also applies to the many staff members of mental health institutions who supervised the use of the book in the initial try-out phase.

We would like to thank Health Insurance Innovation Foundation for the financial contribution that made *Living in the Moment* possible.

We are keen to thank Ando Rokx and Edith Tjoa for their expert and encouraging commentary on the draft version of this book.

A special mention goes to Jurjen Couperus, who diligently processed all of the participants' responses.

Sometimes a picture conveys so much more than words. Our collaboration with Helen van Vliet, who produced the beautiful illustrations in this book, was an added bonus.

A book is always a co-production between authors and publisher. By that token we would like to express our warm gratitude to Elsbeth Greven and Anne Vollaard for their enthusiasm and expert guidance.

We thank Open University Press and Monika Lee in particular for her great commitment and support for this publication and are very grateful to Sue Anderson for her excellent translation of the original Dutch text and finding optimal solutions for many typical Dutch expressions.

About the authors

Ernst Bohlmeijer is a professor at the University of Twente. He has a special interest in narrative psychology, in working with life stories in healthcare and in the role of mindfulness, acceptance and values in promoting mental health. In recent years he has produced a number of publications including *De Verhalen die we Leven* and co-authored the Boom self-help books *Leven met Pijn* and *Op Verhaal Komen*.

Monique Hulsbergen worked for 18 years as a psychologist/ psychotherapist in the mental health sector and is currently working as a freelance psychologist (www.moniquehulsbergen.nl). In 2009 she wrote *Mindfulness – De Aandachtsvolle Therapeut*. In 2010 she co-authored the Boom self-help book *Leven met Pijn*. 2011 and 2012 respectively saw the publication of *Ik ben Altijd Ergens Anders – Over Mindfulness en Leven met Aandacht* and *Emoties, Wat doe Je er Mee?*, also published by Uitgeverij Boom.

Introduction

This book won't teach you how to live a life free from disappointment, pain, gloom, anxiety, doubt and insecurity. Many people experience dissatisfaction with their lives because they are weighed down by problems like these. Only once I've overcome them will I be able to lead the life I want to lead, is the thinking. *A Beginner's Guide to Mindfulness: Live in the Moment* helps you to see and understand that this doesn't work. Trying to avoid mental or physical pain leads to a frenetic effort to lead half a life. In the long term, this intensifies psychological distress. The methods presented in this book are based on acceptance of psychological distress and on increasing psychological flexibility. Acceptance clears the way for living a life with attention, based on your own values. When this works, you experience greater freedom and quality in your life, day after day.

We all have fairy tales read to us as children. Stories that feature princes and princesses having the most thrilling adventures, stories that always end well. The prince meets and rescues the girl of his dreams. The princess is whisked off to a fairy tale castle by her broad-shouldered hero on his pure white steed. And everyone lives happily ever after.

Belief in the 'happy ever after' is deep-rooted. So it's not surprising we put up a fight when life is painful. Life is not easy. Inevitably, there are times when we are full of gloom, doubt, fear, bitter disappointment or insecurity. There are times when the fairy tale is shattered. It's like one of those holidays from the travel brochures. The sea isn't quite so blue, those clouds weren't in the photo, the apartment is a bit of a squeeze and those friendly owners with the beaming smiles are nowhere to be seen. The picture of life that was painted for us was oh-so-enticing, but the reality falls short. We feel cheated. We are living for longer than ever, but permanent happiness continues to elude us.

But then we stir ourselves back into action: surely it can't be as bad as all that? There must be a key to finding happiness. We go in search of the fix that will guarantee a happy ever after. We devour books and courses that promise to make us happy. We do everything we can to rid ourselves of our depression, fears, pain and insecurities. We work ourselves to death. We try every conceivable solution. We trade in our princes and princesses for new ones. We give up drinking. We put on a happy face. And yet, nothing seems to work. The dark clouds just won't disappear, to let us finally start to live our lives. Or perhaps the clouds have finally cleared, we are ready to be happy . . . and then something else comes along: a chronic illness, news of a death, a bad school report, an economic crisis.

So what now?

The problem lies precisely in our opposition to the pain and sorrow in our lives. In this book we propose an alternative approach: *living in the moment*, which has three main cornerstones:

- ➠ Letting go of the fairy tale of 'living happily ever after' (i.e. without pain). Giving up the fight against your psychological distress.
- ➠ Learning to observe what is going on within yourself and to connect with the here and now in your life.
- ➠ Trying to discover what really matters to you in life and making that the basis of your actions.

Why do we believe that this approach helps?

First and foremost, because we ourselves apply these principles in our own daily lives, through all of the ups and downs, and reap the benefits.

Second, due to the enthusiasm expressed by many people

who have tried this method, either individually or in groups. For example, a reader who worked through the book wrote to us:

> *Even now, there are still all sorts of things going on in my life: nice events and really nasty ones. It is as it is. I am present in my life. I'm not losing sight of my values and am using them to do other things as well. I'm still doing the exercises to stay in 'being mode' and to stay kind to myself. I am participating in life.*

And lastly, because scientific research confirms that people benefit from it. Psychological disorders do not disappear, but they do become less intense and shorter in duration. People experience a boost in energy and find their lives more satisfying.

It is important to state that we did not invent the insights and skills presented in this book. Many of them have existed in Eastern cultures for hundreds or even thousands of years. However, in the last three decades these insights and skills have been retailored in clothing more suited to a Western audience.

Jon Kabat-Zinn has taken the longstanding tradition of meditation as practised within Buddhism and presented it in a form more adapted to Western culture: mindfulness. Mindfulness is an important cornerstone of this book.

Steven Hayes and colleagues Kelly Wilson and Kirk Strosahl have introduced a new way of dealing with psychological distress (acceptance rather than opposition) within behaviour therapy: 'acceptance and commitment therapy', or ACT (pronounced 'act') for short. Many of the exercises and insights in this book are based on this method.

However, we believe that the principles of mindfulness and ACT are not valuable simply within a therapeutic context but can also be useful tools to help many more people live satisfying lives. This book is intended as an accessible, step-by-step guide to living life with attention, without fighting psychological distress and based on personal values. A book that inspired us in this respect is *The*

Happiness Trap by Russ Harris, who describes ACT in an accessible manner. A number of the exercises in this book are based on his approach.

A Beginner's Guide to Mindfulness: Live in the Moment is based on two founding principles. Mindfulness and ACT are combined from the start. More so than in existing ACT programmes, we focus systematically on mindfulness throughout the book. And more so than existing mindfulness programmes, this method focuses on becoming aware of opposition, learning how to handle our thoughts and living on the basis of values. The principles of mindfulness and ACT are set out accessibly in a clearly structured programme. We hope that this will enable many people to master the art of *living in the moment* (i.e. with attention and based on values). We have also tried to use accessible examples and language to illustrate the ideas and insights contained in the book.

How to use this book

This book is meant for anyone who is dissatisfied with their life or struggles with psychological distress such as gloom, pain, tiredness, tension, insecurity, fear, listlessness or sadness. It is entirely possible to run through the material in this book by yourself, but if you find this difficult or get stuck, why not get together with someone else who would like to give it a go?

There are three parts to this book. In the first part, you will explore the current methods you use to deal with psychological distress. In the second, you will learn how to give up your fight against psychological distress and learn how to live in 'being mode'. In the third part you will explore the values that matter to you most, and how to live your life based on those values. Learning to observe what is going on within yourself without judging (mindfulness) is a connecting thread that runs through each part of the book. Without conscious awareness, a skill that everyone can develop, it isn't possible to live in the moment.

This book sometimes uses complicated and artificial-sounding terms such as 'cognitive defusion' and 'experiential avoidance'. These terms are in common usage in ACT, so we have chosen to stick with them. You will find explanations of them in a glossary at the end of the book.

Finally, we would like to emphasize one further thing. What this book teaches you is more a way of life than a quick fix or a gimmick. It will probably change your life more than you think, or indeed more than you've initially bargained for. Let us explain what we mean by that: You may already have all sorts of clear-cut goals (expectations) that are part of your personal 'happy ever after' fairy tale. Perhaps you hope this book will teach you some tricks and techniques to help you achieve it. However, we invite you to explore the possibility of starting out with an open mind. Create sufficient space and time in your life. Try to let go of any current goals or expectations you may have, and to treat this as a voyage of discovery. It is then that this book will have the most to offer you.

1

What is 'living in the moment'?

Week 1
What do I want out of life?

Introduction

Isn't there something crazy going on in our Western world? Our standard of living is high. Almost all of us have a roof over our heads, homes that we can heat in the winter. Several times a week we stroll along to the supermarket where we have a choice of 30 kinds of jam, 10 kinds of crisps, 20 washing powders. After our work and chores are done we have a huge variety of television programmes to entertain us. There is no immediate threat of war in the United Kingdom, and a relatively low risk of major natural disasters. What more could we possibly want? And yet, the figures don't lie. Research shows that 25% of adults in the UK (12 million people) suffer from serious psychological disorders such as anxiety and depression. The UK has over two million problem drinkers: not the sort of person who likes a daily glass of wine but people who need to drink in order to function. In the USA, half of all people will seriously contemplate suicide at some time in their lives. Approximately 5% of people attempt suicide at least once in their life. The World Health Organization (WHO) expects depression to become the biggest cause of human suffering within a few decades. Bigger than cancer, Alzheimer's, or any other chronic condition you care to mention. We don't mean to alarm you. Figures are just figures. But if we let them sink in for a moment, they *are* shocking, and we need to ask ourselves what is going wrong.

In material terms, we have never had it so good. We are able to fulfil all of our basic needs in life: food, water, safety and shelter. And yet, many of us are still incapable of leading emotionally satisfying lives. Our own belief is that part of the cause lies in our fanatical pursuit of happiness. We all want that fairy tale 'happy ever after'. And what exactly is wrong with that? Isn't it just a normal human desire?

There are a number of reasons why our desire for happiness can actually make us unhappy.

In the first place, we define happiness as the absence of distress. We seek pleasure and contentment; we want to enjoy ourselves and to avoid disappointment, distress or anger. We have become intolerant of distress. But this is not realistic: distress and its attendant emotions are just as much a part of life as positive emotions. This mindset may have come about because we are capable of so much nowadays, as human beings. We can fly in planes, we have computers, we can create babies in a test tube. We have convinced ourselves that the world can be manipulated. If we can do all of these things, then surely we can make ourselves happy? But that is precisely where we fall short.

Our inner world is much less controllable and open to manipulation than we would like. This makes us even more angry with ourselves, even more distressed, even more anxious and insecure. In a nutshell, our expectations about living a happy life have got out of hand. Happiness is a trap that we dig for ourselves, a trap that we walk into full of hope and expectation, only to clamber out of in disillusionment. Again and again, we seek out different paths to happiness (a new relationship, more money, a different job), but so long as we strive for them without an acceptance of distress, without an acceptance of the less pleasant, darker side of life, without an awareness of our own weaknesses, we will continue to be unhappy.

A second reason is that feelings of happiness are so transient. They are snapshots in time. Once we've finally achieved what we set out to achieve, we *can* experience intense feelings of happiness. But aren't they quick to ebb away again? Don't we come back down to earth within a few days? The paths to happiness can be so long, and the stay there so short.

A third reason for our desire for happiness is that everyone around us *appears* to be so happy. You probably recognize this. In public, everyone puts their best foot forward. They all seem to be doing so well. And if you ask how they are, nearly everyone will respond with an automatic 'Fine, thanks!' We see the fancy cars parked in our neighbours' driveways, we see other happy families out shopping together. And if everyone around us is so happy, we should be able to be happy too. But often, this too turns out to be an illusion. It's all on the outside, it's the external facade that we're so good at maintaining. All sorts of rows, disappointments and pain can be concealed behind the lace curtains. It is deeply ingrained in our culture not to wash our emotional dirty linen in public. But you probably find that when you talk to someone at length, on a deeper level, when you tell them about your struggles, you suddenly meet with signs of recognition. It turns out that most people are struggling and it's not all plain sailing for them either: pain is the rule rather than the exception. Even though, on the outside, it often seems to be the other way round.

A different attitude to mental pain

Happiness, then, is a tricky business. Not that we should be averse to it. Of course not. We should count ourselves very lucky when we *are* happy, and enjoy those moments. But should we pursue happiness so fanatically? That, we're not sure about. Should we simply resign ourselves to the fact that life is not fun? One of the messages of this book is that life becomes more attractive when you stop trying to control your negative emotions, when you give up all of that wrestling with your inner world. Of course, this is easier said than done. It means first of all that – as far as your inner world is concerned – you have to learn to rely less on what your mind tells you. Even though our beloved mind always seems to be our most important ally. We will return to this in more depth later. It also means having to allow and experience all sorts of emotions, rather than fight them, but without giving them full rein. And that can be difficult, because we are so keen to be in control.

But that's not all. Even though we may be setting aside our fanatical pursuit of happiness, we can still pursue an inspired life. 'Inspired' in this context means discovering that anything you do out of inspiration is good. Once we stop investing our energies in trying to control our inner world, we free them up to invest in a meaningful life that is worth living. This book will be your guide as you explore the values that matter most to you; it will invite you to convert those values into plans, and then to put those plans into practice.

Living in the moment

The current prevalence of psychological problems and addictive behaviours appears to show that we have lost our ability to live, the 'art of living', to some extent. In our view, the art of living is the ability to live in the moment. Living in the moment means being open to and accepting both positive and negative emotions. Living in the moment encompasses both happiness and distress. When we try to avoid negative emotions and distress, our psychological flexibility is diminished. Our actions become more frenetic and our 'room for living' shrinks. Living in the moment also means figuring out an answer to the question of what makes life worth living for us. It means knowing what our most important values are, so that we can set priorities and not be so easily daunted by setbacks. Living in the moment means actively imparting meaning to life and living based on vitality, living from the heart. Living in the moment is not living on the basis of YES, BUT. . . or IF. . . THEN. . . . It is living on the basis of BOTH. . . AND. Yes, we may be gloomy, stressed and insecure but we are also getting on with what matters to us. Living in the moment means giving it your best, 'going for it'. Living in the moment means being able to avoid looking back on your life with regret and thinking 'if only I'd. . .'.

A satisfying life

This book provides tools to help you rediscover the art of living, so you can start to live a more satisfying life. The method we use is based on ACT and mindfulness. ACT stands for *acceptance and commitment therapy*, a method developed in the United States by Steven Hayes and colleagues. Mindfulness is the ability to observe what is going on in yourself, without judging. Originally a concept from Buddhism, mindfulness has been made accessible to a Western audience by authors such as Jon Kabat-Zinn.

Six skills are central to this book, each of which will be discussed at length later on.

1 *Acceptance.* You start by working on your readiness to experience psychological distress. Through a series of exercises, you gain an understanding that strategies focused on avoiding or controlling don't work and may even be counterproductive (in that they don't contribute to the life you want to lead). You learn to tolerate situations and emotions that you currently try to avoid.

2 *Cognitive defusion.* You learn that avoidance is usually caused by your thoughts about life experiences and emotions. The aim is not so much to replace these thoughts with others (this is not effective in the long term) as to distance yourself from them, to see thoughts as thoughts and not as reality, by refusing to identify with them. In ACT, this is known as cognitive defusion.

3 *Mindfulness.* You learn to become aware of your experiences in the here and now. This is necessary in order to gain an awareness of automatic response patterns. Being present with your full attention in the here and now increases your flexibility and inner peace. In time, you will become kinder to yourself and those around you. You will start to experience greater freedom of choice.

4 *The observing self.* As you gain experience of mindfulness, you

will begin to realize that you are more than the sum of your thoughts and emotions. You are the ever-present ability to experience. In ACT, this is called the observing self.

5   *Values.* You spend time examining the values that are important to you in life. You learn how to make those values the compass by which you live.

6   *Values in practice.* You translate your values into concrete actions and steps. As you start to live increasingly according to your values, your life becomes ever fuller and more satisfying.

At this point you may still be scratching your head in bewilderment, and some of the terms used will sound strange to you. But this book sets out to explain everything step by step and will give you plenty of opportunities to practise. Anyone can learn these skills. You don't need to be convinced at this stage, but we do hope, of course, that we have piqued your curiosity. Bear with us: we are about to try your patience for a little while longer. Over the next few weeks you will start by exploring what you have done so far to overcome your pain and distress, and what the results have been.

Exercise: the 'backpack of sorrows'

In this exercise (based on Hayes 2005) we ask you to list all the things that are bothering you, the things you are wrestling with in your life at present. This exercise is about emotions, feelings, thoughts, habits and behaviours you'd like to rid yourself of. In a sense, it's about the painful baggage that you lug around with you, all day, every day. It's about your burden or 'backpack' of sorrows. Here are some examples:

> I am sad about my grandmother's death.
> I have a short temper.
> I eat too much.
> I can't face getting up in the mornings.

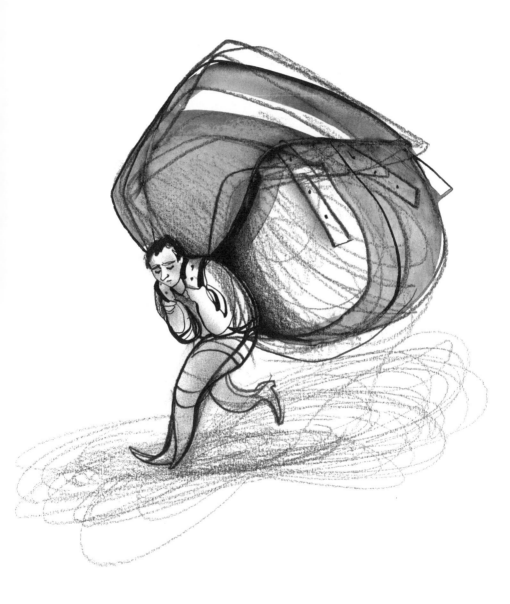

> ❯ I feel guilty about not spending enough time with my children.
> ❯ I feel worthless.
> ❯ I feel exhausted.
> ❯ I feel insecure.
> ❯ I drink too much.
> Etc.

Things that bother me	For how long?

After you've made the list, write after each item for how long this emotion or behaviour has been bothering you.

Now we would like you to redo the list, this time putting the items in order, with the thing that bothers you most at the top and the thing that bothers you least at the bottom.

Bothers me most	To what extent does it stop you leading the life you want to lead (1 = only a little; 10 = totally)? For how long?
....	....
....	....
....	....
....	....
....	....
....	....
....	....
....	....
....	....

Once you've done this, you can write after each item the extent to which the feeling, thought or behaviour stops you leading the life you would like to lead.

This list is probably one of the main reasons you bought this book and set to work with it. You have hauled all of your psychological sorrows out of the backpack and spread them out in front of you. This is the current state of affairs, before you made a start on this book. If only the solution were so simple as putting your baggage down beside you and just walking away. This would be a slim volume if it were! But the backpack of psychological sorrows is firmly in place on our shoulders. And the painful items just keep slipping in there. They are there when we go to bed, and they are there when we get up. You probably feel it is this backpack, or some of the items in it, that are obstructing your freedom of movement, holding you back from living in the moment. Over the next 2 weeks you will start to explore how you handle these 'sorrows'. And by the end of the book you should see some changes in the list.

Exercise: the 'miracle question'

But now imagine that you wake up tomorrow, and each day after that, and the backpack of sorrows has miraculously grown a bit lighter. The five heaviest items, your top five psychological sorrows, have disappeared. Take a moment to let that sink in.

Then answer the following questions for each item from the top five. The most important thing is to state how – in what respect – the quality of your life would change. It is about saying what you would do that really matters to you.

Some examples:

> If I weren't so anxious, I'd want to see much more of the world and learn more about different cultures.
> If I didn't have such an urge to perform well, I'd be able to enjoy my work more.
> If I weren't so insecure, I'd be able to have a meaningful relationship.

If it weren't for ....

I would ....

If it weren't for ....

I would ....

If it weren't for ....

I would ....

1

If it weren't for ....

I would ....

If it weren't for ....

I would ....

You have now put into words what 'living in the moment' means to you: how you would live if you were free of anxiety, insecurity, anger, doubt, sadness and so on. If nothing much occurs to you at the moment, that's fine. We expect that over the next few weeks you'll become more aware of what you would do if you weren't held back by your 'sorrows'.

Metaphor: the landscape of living in the moment

Your ideas about living in the moment, about the ideal life you'd like to lead, could be seen as a map of your life marked out with scenic routes. Perhaps there are also some clear landmarks showing the direction you want to take: a distant hill or mountain, a church steeple in a village, a stream you could walk along for a while. You are able to follow these routes if you keep your attention on the map and your surroundings. But there's always that heavy backpack weighing you down as well. And the backpack contains all those different items vying for your attention, so you can't focus it where it is needed.
   Reflection:

⇒ What would that map look like for you?
⇒ What routes would you want to follow?
⇒ What landmarks are showing you the way?

1

Example

Iris suffers from panic attacks that are making her life hell. Anything that is new, she avoids. The attacks started after her father died, 8 years ago. It was an awful period and she understands now that she felt miserable at the time. She has already tried a variety of options in a bid to shake off the attacks: seeing a psychologist, medication, acupuncture. Nothing has helped to get the attacks under control and she has become despondent. She tots up how much time and money she has spent in her quest to conquer her panic attacks.

The panic attacks are at number one on her list of sorrows. Asked what she would do if a miracle were to intervene and the panic attacks were to melt away like snow in the midday sun, she tells the following story. She'd always been an independent-minded woman, who loved travelling and meeting people: the unexpected. She was curious to know what life would be like without the panic attacks. For a long time now, she has wanted to go on a trip to South America. Every year the travel brochure arrives in the post and she's gradually starting to think nothing will ever come of it. 'If it weren't for the panic attacks I'd be on the first plane to Lima and the adventure could begin', she says.

Eternal recurrence

Friedrich Nietzsche was a famous German philosopher who lived from 1844 to 1900. You might call him the philosopher of 'living in the moment'. He wrote at length about the art of living, about dealing with pain and about the art of enjoying life. Nietzsche knew what he was talking about: he suffered frequently from depression in the course of his life.

In his books, he constantly incites people to live in the moment. For example, in *The Gay Science*, he wrote: 'What if a demon were to creep after you one night, in your loneliest loneliness, and say, "This life which you live must be lived by you once again and innumerable times more; and every pain and joy and thought and sigh must come again to you, all in the same sequence. The eternal hourglass will again and again be turned and you with it, dust of the dust!"'

The film *Groundhog Day*, with Bill Murray in the leading role, has this as a central theme. The vital question we can ask ourselves is: 'How would we feel if the rest of our life was exactly the same as what had gone before?' If you can answer 'Great!' whole-heartedly, you know you're living in the moment. But if your answer is 'I don't want to think about it', or if you're not sure, you know there's work to be done and that you probably didn't pick up this book without good reason.

Mindfulness exercise: the body scan

One of the most important skills for 'living in the moment' is mindfulness. Mindfulness is the ability to notice what is going on within yourself, and how you respond to it, without judging. Mindfulness is so important because it helps you to discover automatic, unconscious patterns in your life. You can't make changes in your life until you're aware of the way you're living now. And with mindfulness, you can also enhance your own intuition and innate wisdom: your body and heart often give clues to what you think about something, and you learn to pick up those clues.

Mindfulness is learned mainly through meditation exercises, translated for the Western world primarily by Jon Kabat-Zinn. The exercises in this book are based on this. It is a skill that takes a lot of practice at the start, and you may also experience an initial threshold of resistance or restlessness. It's all part and parcel of the process. If you want to create a beautiful garden, you will first have to clear away a lot of weeds. But you will notice that it becomes easier and easier and more natural over time.

1

In this exercise you learn to observe the sensations occurring in your body. In a sense, you 'take the pulse' of each part of the body by bringing your attention to it. With frequent practice, you learn to notice more effectively (and more quickly) what is going on within you, how you feel, how you respond to what you are experiencing. In the long term, this enables you to break out of automatic patterns of response.

This exercise lasts for around 17 minutes. Practise every day over the coming week. Choose a quiet time. Make any arrangements you need to with family or friends to ensure that you are not disturbed during that time. Set an alarm to go off after the practice.

The essence of the exercise is to bring your attention in turn (at a calm and steady pace) to your left foot, left lower leg, left knee, left thigh, *whole left leg,* right foot, right lower leg, right knee, right thigh, *whole right leg,* your hips, pubic area, stomach, chest, back, *whole torso,* left hand, left forearm, left elbow, left upper arm, *whole left arm,* right hand, right forearm, right elbow, right upper arm, *whole right arm,* throat, neck, back of the head, forehead, nose and mouth, jaw, *whole head.* Then you focus your awareness on your whole body (see Appendix on page 19 for a more detailed version of the short body scan).

The aim of the exercise is not to relax, but to notice what is there. The sensations you experience may be pleasant, unpleasant or neutral.

If you find your mind is wandering (perhaps distracted by a stray thought or a noise), simply notice that, and bring your attention gently back to your body.

Stop and think

You are now a little better acquainted with this book about 'living in the moment'. Its aim is to help you create a life that is no longer centred around fighting psychological pain, but around shaping your values. But now is a good time to linger for a moment and ask yourself a couple of questions. We don't want you to drop out disappointed in a few weeks' time; that would be a shame, and a waste of your time and energy.

Do I really want this?

Are you sufficiently motivated to make any drastic changes that may be needed in your life? Do you want to make space in your life for change? You can test this yourself by checking if you have made time over the past week for this book and the exercises. Are you prepared at this point in time to give up activities in your life in order to do the exercises in this book? You may have good reasons for not proceeding any further right now. Maybe you're happy enough with your life as it is. Maybe you don't want to give up any activities in your life at this time. Maybe you were hoping for quick solutions to certain problems in your life. Maybe your main reason for trying the book was a problem in your life that seems to be resolving itself. If that's the case, you might want to consider setting the book aside for now and perhaps picking it up again at a later date.

Do I want to look at myself?

This book has a purpose and a point, *if* you are prepared to examine your own behaviour and opportunities. But if you are still focused on being angry with people and circumstances around you, and are set on changing them, it may make sense to try that first. And if that doesn't work, the question remains: are you prepared to look at your own part in your problems?

What are my experiences of learning?

We suggest taking a moment to think about your experiences of learning up until now. What sort of person were you at school? What new things have you learned in recent years? What is your approach to learning? Are you patient, or do you give up quickly? There are new skills to be learnt in this book as well. By thinking about your experiences of learning to date, and your approach to learning, you may be able to identify patterns more quickly in the coming weeks. And when you identify those patterns, you may be able to approach them differently if necessary.

Write down some of your experiences with learning to date.

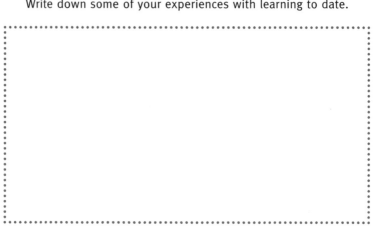

Appendix: short body scan

In the following exercise, you will focus your attention on your body in a friendly way. Scan your body from head to toe. Acknowledge all the experiences you encounter, and try to allow them as much as possible. Don't expect that you'll be able to keep your attention constantly focused on this exercise. In the exercise, parts of the body are mentioned, such as your arms, legs and head. The intention is to carry out a quick status check on the part of the body that is mentioned; spend 6–10 seconds on that part of the body before reading on.

➡ Sit on a straight-backed chair with your legs parallel and your feet on the floor. If you feel comfortable, close your eyes.

➡ Notice what is to the forefront at this moment. There might be a variety of thoughts; there might be a particular feeling, such as tension, boredom or irritation; you might feel curious. Notice and acknowledge what is there at this moment.

➡ Feel the way your body makes contact with the chair you are sitting on. Notice which parts of the body are supported and where you feel contact with the chair and the floor.

➡ Take your attention to your left leg and left foot. Focus your attention on the whole of your left leg and foot. Notice what you encounter. If you don't feel anything, that's OK. Or you may feel a sense of relaxation, or tension, pain, warmth or cold. Acknowledge and notice what is there at this moment.

➡ Now take your attention to your right leg and right foot.

⇒ Focus your attention on the whole of your right leg and foot.

⇒ Focus your attention on both legs.

During this exercise, your attention will wander sooner or later. You may have started thinking. Perhaps you're becoming tense or impatient. Wandering off is normal and only human. When you *notice* that you've wandered off, you are present in the now again, and you go back to scanning your body.

⇒ Let go of the focus on your legs and take your attention to your torso. Pay attention to your hips. . ., pelvis. . ., back. . ., stomach. . . and chest. . . Acknowledge and notice what you perceive. Embrace your whole torso with your attention.

⇒ Now take your attention to your shoulders. This is an area where tension can build up. Pay attention to this area in a friendly way. Try not to change anything. Allow the feeling.

⇒ Now take your attention to your left hand and left arm. Notice if you perceive anything here. If you don't perceive anything, that's OK. You may feel tingling, warmth or cold, tension or pain. Allow what is there.

⇒ Take your attention to your right hand and right arm. Focus your attention on the whole of your right arm.

⇒ Focus your attention on both arms.

⇒ Take your attention to your throat and neck. Notice what you encounter. Whatever you encounter, it's OK. You don't need to change anything.

1

⟼ Now take your attention to your head and face. Notice what you feel in the back of your head, on top of your head, in your forehead and face.

⟼ Expand your attention to your whole body. Don't focus on a specific place. Be aware of the physical perceptions in your body at this moment.

⟼ And now you can bring the exercise to an end by opening your eyes and having a stretch.

Week 2
I'm not here (at the moment)

The only drama there is,
is not wanting the experience we are having.
Isaac Shapiro

Introduction

1

Last week you thought about what makes life worth living for you.
We also talked about the pursuit of happiness as a trap. By
chasing happiness, we are actually seeking only half a life. We
want to feel good, cheerful, proud, satisfied. Ideally, we'd like
every day to be a holiday. We don't want sadness, pain,
desolation, gloom, fear, disappointment. We want life, but not
death. We want youth, not old age. We only want half a life. We'd
like nothing better than to stop the sun and earth in their tracks at
the height of summer, when the days are long and warm, people
are generally more cheerful and life feels more carefree. But that's
not the way it works. The earth keeps turning and, before you
know it, the days are getting shorter, colder and wetter. Autumn
and winter are just as much a part of life as spring and summer.

And as it is with the seasons, so it is with our inner world. We
want the lovely, bright side of life, not the ugly, darker side. And
we do our utmost to achieve it. We try with all our might to stop
the earth from turning. We try to get our negative emotions under
control. Or we try to escape and just not be there. Our attempts to
avoid the dark side of life have significant consequences: they only
worsen the pain. Slowly but surely, we slip into a waking slumber,
in winter and summer alike.

In Week 1 you made a list of types of distress or 'sorrows': a summary of the emotions and situations that you are struggling with and that led you to buy this book. This is the distress in your life that you want to get rid of; the pain you want to avoid. There are a number of options. Broadly speaking, we use three strategies to avoid experiencing negative emotions: prevention, distraction and relief.

⇢ *Prevention.* This strategy focuses on avoiding situations that cause the distress. If work exhausts us, we stop going to work. If open spaces make us anxious or afraid, we stop going out.

⇢ *Distraction.* The distraction strategy focuses on diverting our thoughts and feelings, pretending the pain isn't there. If we feel empty inside, we throw ourselves into our work. If we feel bad, we try to think about something nice.

⇢ *Relief.* This strategy focuses on blotting out our distress, on numbing our pain. If we are hurting, we swallow pills. If we come home stressed out, we drink a few glasses of something alcoholic. If we feel glum, we munch our way through a bag of crisps or a packet of biscuits. Or we slump in front of the television all evening.

Experiential avoidance

What are we actually doing when we apply the strategies outlined above? We are trying to avoid experiencing what we're experiencing at that moment. We can't bear our emotions so we try to evade them, fix our attention on something else, or anaesthetize them. We pretend the pain of that moment isn't there. It is as if we are pulling the plug on life. Sadness, fear, pain, disappointment or emptiness come knocking on our door but we don't let them in, we pretend we're not at home. In psychology and ACT this is known as 'experiential avoidance'. 'Experiential' derives from 'experience'. We avoid experiencing what happens to us.

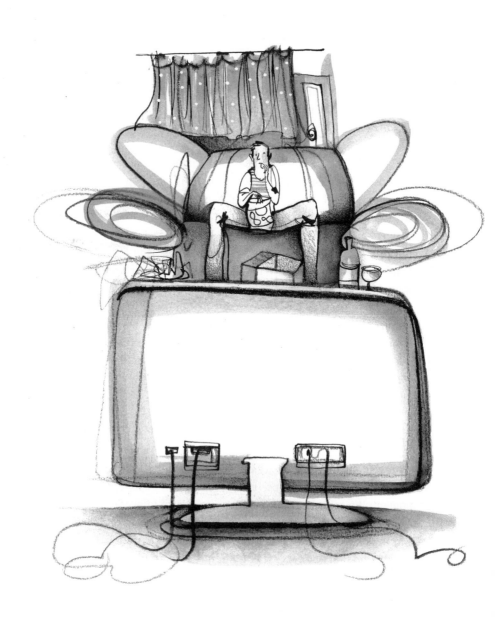

The strategies we use to avoid distress have something very attractive about them at first sight. They work! When we avoid putting ourselves in situations that make us anxious, we don't feel anxious any more. When we scoff a packet of biscuits, we dull the sharp edge of our anger. When we avoid seeing our brother or sister, we don't experience that sibling conflict any more. When we open a bottle or smoke a couple of cigarettes, life is suddenly appealing again. When we swallow a pill, the pain recedes. Great. What's wrong with that?

However, there are a number of reasons why experiential avoidance is not effective in the long term.

The first reason is that experiential avoidance is a short-term fix. It helps for a few hours, maybe a day, but after that nothing has changed. The pain comes back, just as sharp as before. And in the long run we have to do even more (eat more, pop more pills, drink more) to suppress the pain. In that respect, avoidance is like scratching an itch. Scratching an insect bite helps for a while, but then the itch comes back all the stronger. Hence, the common observation in ACT that 'the solution is the problem'.

Avoidance can lead to more pain in two ways.

1   Avoidance leads to a short-term reduction in pain. In the long term, you will have to do more and more to suppress it, which may lead to more and more avoidance. The effects tend to snowball.

Jack is afraid of crowds in enclosed spaces. When his friends invite him out to the cinema, he turns them down because he wants to avoid the stress the outing will entail. And the next time, when they go to London for a day, he doesn't go with them. In the long run, they stop asking. Slowly but surely, Jack's friends drift away and increasingly he finds himself at home alone. Now he has another worry: that his friends find him wet and boring. So he doesn't try to make any new friends either, and becomes more and more isolated.

2 Avoidance can have a negative effect on the way you think about yourself. Because the pain increases, you have to devise more and more strategies to keep it numbed.

Karen is having problems at work and doesn't feel appreciated. When she comes home, she launches straight into the wine. In time, one glass becomes two and two becomes three. Her sleep is affected and she never feels rested any more. She starts to call in sick from time to time. Sitting at home, she feels inadequate and fed up with herself. So her drinking starts earlier and earlier.

1

And perhaps the most important thing is that avoidance doesn't bring us any closer to a life worth living. On the contrary, it takes us further away. Hayes (2005) calls this the pain of *absence*. Avoidance leads us to invest energy in behaviour that is aimed at blotting out the pain. As a result, we are no longer focused on what really matters to us in life. If our main preoccupation is with lightening the burden of our 'backpack of sorrows', we are not following the routes we want to take. We are living a more and more restricted life. Half a life becomes a quarter, a quarter becomes an eighth. We have less pain (in the short term), but we're also experiencing less, enjoying less, meeting fewer people, challenging ourselves less. And in the long term, that starts to cause pain too! When we try to avoid the pain that is part of life (also called 'clean' pain; Hayes et al. 1999), it will only increase and spread to other areas (this is also called 'dirty' pain).

Are avoidance strategies always bad?

No, not necessarily. It can't do any harm to leave things as they are once in a while, for an evening or a weekend, and to submerge ourselves in intoxication and oblivion. We all need to pull the plug sometimes. If we can then face up to our distress again, and experience and express it, there's no problem. That's why the title of this chapter includes 'at the moment' in brackets. Avoidance is ineffective, and even harmful, chiefly when it becomes a pattern in our lives, when we're absent more often than we are present. Scientific research demonstrates convincingly that experiential avoidance, in the long term, has extremely negative effects on our health.

Conclusion

Our fanatical attempts to live half a life, to experience the emotions of spring and summer but not those of autumn and winter, have significant drawbacks. They lead to not living at all. Half a life is no life. It takes us away from, rather than closer to, the landmarks in the landscape of the life that we would like to lead. Once you understand and gradually face up to this, and once you start to see that experiential avoidance is constraining your life, you have already taken an important step on the road towards a rich and meaningful life that is worth living.

Your favourite avoidance strategies

The focus of this task is on experiential avoidance: all the things we do to avoid psychological pain, or to avoid experiencing it. Write down some of your favourite avoidance strategies (Hayes et al. 1999). To help start you off, we have given you a number of examples.

Prevention	Distraction	Relief
Not going out	Watching television	Drinking
Avoiding enclosed spaces	Going clothes shopping	Smoking
Avoiding certain people	Denial (pretending it doesn't exist)	Snacking

Write down your favourite avoidance strategies.

1

2

3

4

5

6

7

8

9

10

The results

The next task is for you to complete the following list. In the left-hand column, one beneath the other, write down the avoidance strategies you have just described. Now think about each of these strategies for a moment. Try to remember when you used the strategy in the past few weeks. And then answer the following questions for each strategy.

1 Was your behaviour effective in the short term? In other words, did it help you to reduce the pain, to avoid it, to blot it out? You can answer yes, moderately or no. Write your answer in the second column.

2 Was your behaviour effective in the long term? Did it cause the pain to disappear from your life over time, or did it greatly reduce it? Overall, have you become less insecure, anxious, isolated, etc.? Again, you can answer yes, moderately or no. Write your answer in the third column.

3 Finally, we ask you to consider your life the way you'd like to lead it, the way you described it in the 'miracle question' exercise. The question now is whether the strategy you apply helps you achieve this. For each behaviour in the left-hand column, ask yourself if it has brought you closer to the life you'd like to lead. You can answer yes, moderately or no. Note down your answers in the right-hand column.

Avoidance behaviour	Effective in short term?	Effective in long term?	Brought you closer to living in the moment?
1			
2			
3			
4			
5			
6			

....

....

7

....

8

....

9

....

10

————— ————— ————— ————— —————

Once you've completed this list, take a look at your answers. What conclusion do you come to?

1

....

....

....

....

....

....

....

Diary of painful moments

Over the next week we would like you to keep a diary of your avoidance behaviour – without trying to change it! Every day, describe a moment or event that caused you to experience psychological pain. First, give a brief description of the situation. Then write down your emotions and feelings. Finally, describe your behaviour.

A couple of examples are given to start you off.

Monday

Situation	11 am. My mother rang up and had a moan.
Emotion/feeling	I felt angry and responsible, as if it's my fault.
Behaviour	I went shopping and bought a load of clothes.

Tuesday

Situation	5.30 pm. I was in the car on the way home. There was a traffic jam.
Emotion/feeling	Tired, agitated.
Behaviour	I ate a whole bag of sweets.

Monday

Situation

Emotion/feeling

Behaviour

Tuesday

Situation

Emotion/feeling

Behaviour

Wednesday

Situation

Emotion/feeling

Behaviour

Thursday

Situation

Emotion/feeling

Behaviour

Friday

Situation

Emotion/feeling

Behaviour

Saturday

Situation

Emotion/feeling

Behaviour

Sunday

Situation

Emotion/feeling

Behaviour

This is an important awareness-raising exercise. It helps you to become aware of situations that cause you stress, and how you currently handle that. At the end of the week, take a look back at your diary. Do certain things catch your eye? Are there certain avoidance strategies that you didn't know you had? What is the emotion you experience most often?

1

Metaphor: the unwelcome guest

Imagine you're organizing a party for the whole family. You want to make it a big event, and everyone's invited. But the family has a black sheep, in the shape of Uncle John. John stinks to high heaven, always eats half the food and talks with his mouth full. And he only has one topic of conversation – the fact that he used to captain a cargo ship – so everyone finds him hard going. Not only that, but he's big, tough and fairly antisocial. Ideally, you'd rather not invite John, but he always knows when there are family parties in the offing and has a tendency to 'drop by on the spur of the moment'. Can you picture the scenario?

How are you going to handle this situation? You really don't want John to come and 'spoil' your party. This means spending a nervous few days worrying about whether he'll show up, and how you will handle that. On the evening itself, you hover near the door, keeping a constant watch to see if Uncle John is on his way. And when he finally appears, he won't be sent away ('I'll just stay for a short while'). Then you're constantly running after him to check that he's not annoying anyone and not shovelling the whole cake on to his plate.

Before you read any further, take a minute to let this picture sink in. This unwelcome guest may stand for everything in your life that you're fighting against. Do you recognize this as a picture of where you are in life? Do you recognize the need to control everything? What are the consequences for yourself?

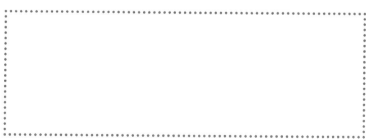

Continue to page 42.

Mindfulness: the past week

Over the past week you have been practising the body scan. Write down some of the things you have experienced.

1

Experience shows that some people find meditation pleasant and helpful from the outset, but others find it difficult. The main thing is not to lose courage. Bear in mind that you are learning a new skill that takes time. A number of frequently asked questions are addressed below. The answers may help you to do the exercises.

I can only keep the exercise up for a short time. What now?
At the outset, sitting still for 5 minutes can be a lot to ask. The important thing is to keep practising every day. Even if it's only 5 minutes, that's 5 minutes well spent. It can sometimes help to ask yourself why you can't keep it up, what's stopping you? For example, if you're feeling very stressed or restless, you can respond to that by bringing the practice to an end.

You can also put a name to the way you are feeling as you do the exercise. Keep saying to yourself 'restless, restless, restless, etc.' or 'stressed, stressed, stressed, etc.' or 'impatient, impatient,

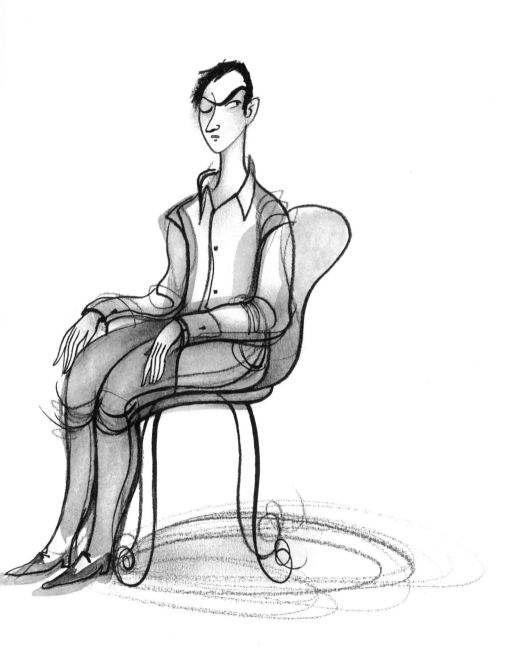

impatient, etc.'. Notice where you perceive this in your body. Try not to fight it, but embrace the feeling in your body with your attention, in a friendly, non-judgemental way. Let it be. Perhaps then you can slowly increase the length of the exercise.

I'm not managing to do the exercise. My thoughts keep wandering.

How do you know that you're constantly drifting? You must have noticed it! That means you're doing the exercise right. It's about noticing what is going on now, in the foreground. If that is thinking, it is thinking. When you *notice* that you're thinking, you stop living on automatic pilot. It's also important, therefore, not to condemn yourself for all that thinking. Notice it, stay kind towards yourself, and continue with the body scan in a friendly way. And, who knows, perhaps the thinking *will* diminish at some stage.

I don't have any time to do the exercises.

We need to get strict here for a minute. Not having time is a choice. It means that you haven't been prepared to make any time for the exercises so far. That can mean two things. Either you're not prepared to free up any time. Perhaps because you're already happy enough with your life as it is, and feel good in yourself. If that's the case, you might consider calling it a day with this book. Or you need to make a 'painful' choice by giving up something else. Take a close look at all the things that occupy your time. Do you really find all of these activities satisfying? Do you give everything your full attention? Probably not, or you wouldn't have started this book. Isn't there something you could drop? What does that leave you with, for a more satisfying life?

1

Mindfulness exercise: observing the breath

This week you are going to practise a new meditation exercise. In it, you follow your breath as it happens from moment to moment. The intention is not to change, direct or control the breath. Some breathing exercises aim to deepen the breath, for example. That is not the intention here. If it happens, it's OK; if it doesn't happen, that's OK too. This exercise is purely about following the breath as it is. Following your breath can serve as an anchor to ground you in the now.

Sit on a straight-backed chair, with your back against the chair back, your legs out parallel in front of you and your feet on the floor. Make sure you are wearing loose clothing, especially around the waist. This is an alert, wide-awake position, in which you can develop attentiveness.

Notice first of all how you are sitting on the chair. There may be all sorts of thoughts running through your mind, there may be a particular feeling, are there any physical sensations, are you curious or tense? Notice that, and acknowledge what you are feeling at this moment. Feel the contact between your body and the chair (back, hips and thighs). Then notice where you perceive your breathing most obviously. You can feel the breath in your nostrils, where you can sense cool air coming in and warmed air going out. You can also follow the breath by directing your attention to the rise and fall of your chest or abdomen. Choose the place where you find it easiest to follow the breath.

Then follow your breathing for a while (e.g. 8–15 minutes). A useful aid is to count each out-breath. Especially at the start, this enables you to keep your attention focused on the breath more easily. Counting is an aid; it is not about how high you can count. Any time you lose track, just go back to one and start again. Be kind to yourself, it's not a competition.

Your attention is bound to wander more than once. This is normal, and only human. The attention can be caught by all sorts of thoughts (planning, judging, worrying, analysing, remembering, etc.). It can also drift due to physical perceptions, of pain or an itch for example. The mind can also wander due to certain feelings, such as sadness, joy, desire, fear, stress or impatience. Noises or other stimuli can also carry you away.

If you notice that you've wandered off, simply note where your attention is. Then, in a friendly way, direct it back to the breath. Wandering off is not a bad thing. In fact, by noticing it, you are developing your awareness of what is happening from moment to moment.

When the practice is over, observe the effect it has had on you. If you feel relieved, take note of this. Perhaps you're surprised how fast the time has gone. If so, note this too.

1

A frozen heart

Dutch-born author and speaker Jan Bommerez wrote a book about 'flow', a process that was described by the psychologist Mihaly Csikszentmihalyi as a process of total immersion in an activity. It means going with the flow of life. Clarity, choice, centredness, connection, challenge and confidence are the preconditions required for flow. Jan Bommerez raises the possibility of adding a seventh 'C': 'congruence', which means remaining true to your values and principles.

The main obstacle to flow is a frozen heart: 'The deepest pain, the hardest core in our closed personality is our lost trust in the fundamental 'goodness' of life. That is what is meant by loss of innocence. This loss makes us defensive and calculating. Due to this deeply suppressed pain, we start to live more and more in order to avoid things, rather than in order to express our individuality joyfully through creative action.' (Bommerez 2007, p. 205)

Thawing your heart begins with re-allowing and re-experiencing your psychological pain.

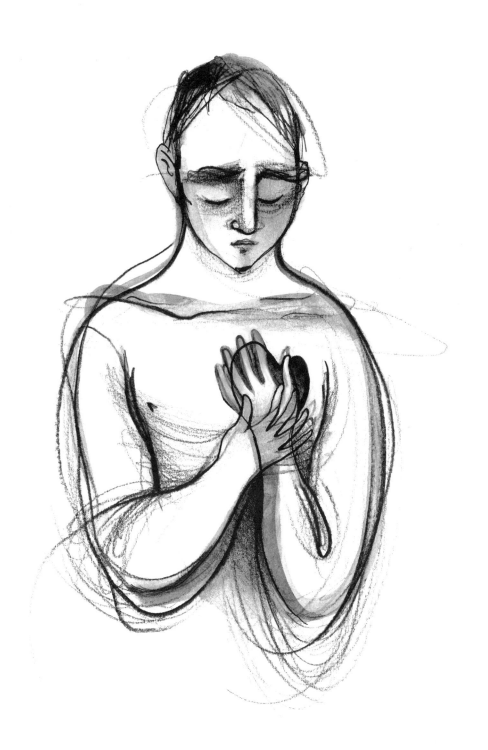

Metaphor: the unwelcome guest (continued)

Do you recognize the way that your own attitude allows the unwelcome guest to ruin the atmosphere, both in the run-up and during the party? You can't simply relax, look forward to the party and enjoy it. You're too busy trying to manage and control the situation.

You could also decide to let it go. If he comes, he comes. The guests will just have to deal with him themselves, and there will probably be enough food to go round. You focus your full attention on the party. What is the effect? You enjoy the party *and* you bump into John from time to time.

Now return to page 35.

1

Week 3
Leave your mind out of it

You cannot direct the winds
but you can adjust the sails.
Jon Kabat-Zinn

Introduction

Last week you thought about the methods we often use to get control over our inner selves (mainly over pain and unpleasant feelings): prevention, distraction and relief. It has probably become clear to you that, although these methods may work in the short term, in the long term they don't solve the problem and may even make it worse. Another common method is using the mind to try to control our feelings, which seems to be a good choice. After all, our mind is our most important survival mechanism, isn't it? Haven't we been told to use our 'brain' or our 'common sense' more than once in our lives?

Without our ability to reflect, we would still be living in prehistoric times and indeed might not have survived at all as a species. Many animals are physically stronger than humans, and better protected against a variety of natural conditions. Camels are able to store large quantities of water and can therefore survive in the desert for long periods. A polar bear's coat is so thick it can withstand conditions at the North Pole.

But it is we humans who have become the dominant species on Earth, for which we have our minds to thank! We are able to plan and think logically. As a result, we have learnt to farm crops and animals, to build houses, to make clothes. All of which makes us less dependent on the whims of nature. We have learnt to print books, allowing us to store information and to distribute it more quickly, so we are no longer dependent on oral tradition. And think of all the things we can do in the twenty-first century! Fly in a plane, send e-mails, preserve food, live into old age, to name but a few.

We are able to solve problems, to control our environment, thanks to our ability to reflect logically and to analyse. THINKING = CONTROL. Given this power of the mind, it is only logical that we should try to control the way we feel through intellectual reflection. But does the mind help in this respect?

There are many exercises that show that thinking gives us little control over our inner world. Try for a couple of minutes, as hard as you can, not to think of a pink elephant. There's a good chance that the opposite will happen, that you will spend the whole time thinking of a pink elephant. Sometimes it works for a while, but then the pink elephant reappears in all its glory. Or imagine you are flying in a plane and the engines on one side fail, causing the aircraft to lurch violently. The pilot makes an announcement over the intercom to reassure passengers there is nothing to be afraid of. This advice may help to stop you panicking, but the idea won't stop most people being afraid.

What is striking about this is that the feelings we try to suppress come to the fore all the more strongly. It's like trying to push a ball under water. However hard you push, the ball springs back again as soon as you stop. It is, in fact, the mind that urges us to suppress feelings. Three processes are at play here: the content of our thinking, the fusing of thoughts with who we are and our power of imagination.

Content of our thinking: evaluative and compelling thoughts

Thoughts that have the greatest influence on how we feel have certain characteristics: they are 'evaluative' (judging) or 'compelling'. Evaluative thoughts are thoughts that involve a judgement about a situation or about ourselves. In a way, we are sticking a label on a situation. Compelling thoughts are thoughts that involve imposing something on ourselves, wanting something from ourselves. Evaluative and compelling thoughts are often seamlessly intertwined.

A few examples:

Evaluative thoughts	Compelling thoughts
Crying is wrong, men shouldn't cry.	Stop crying.
I feel insecure, and I mustn't.	I need to be strong.
I'm a scaredy-cat.	Don't be such a baby.
Am I still grieving? I should be over it by now.	Get a grip on yourself.
I feel lousy, I'm such a loser.	Stop overreacting.

These thoughts can be so fleeting and so automatic that we are not even aware of them.

Fusing thoughts and reality

Thoughts have often become so natural to us that we view them as reality: as if they are experience itself. *I'm worthless* is a thought (a judgement) about certain experiences, but we can identify so closely with this thought that we experience it as real. We no longer perceive it as thought, but as reality.

In ACT, this is called 'cognitive fusion'. Thoughts that pass judgement on ourselves as people have a particular effect on our identity, so they also have a strong influence on the way we feel.

Power of imagination

The power of imagination is very strong. Imagine that you are biting into a lemon. You may find your jaw moving of its own accord. We can take this power of imagination and apply it positively, looking back on our lives, reflecting on what we have experienced. In principle, therefore, we can learn from our mistakes. And we can also think ahead. We are able to link imaginary situations and actions, which enables us to devise solutions, for example: 'If I do X first, and then Y, assuming Z at the same time, it'll work.'

However, we often apply our power of imagination in a negative sense. We brood over the past: 'Why did it have to be that way? If only I'd done X, then. . .' Sports stars are often heard to say that they replayed a game or match over and over in their heads the night after losing it.

Likewise, all kinds of disaster scenarios for the future arise *in our thoughts*. We fret and worry about all the things that *could* go wrong. And we believe firmly in the reality of those thoughts, because otherwise they wouldn't cause us such distressing feelings (anxiety, depression, inferiority, hopelessness).

The vital feature of all of these processes is that we don't take the experience as it is but seek to control it using the power of the mind. We don't want to feel insecure, afraid, tired, gloomy, guilty or frustrated, so we try to bend life to our will using our minds. Once again, the mind is a great help in dealing with external problems but is often a bad counsellor when it comes to emotional problems.

Our ideal would be to revise our past, to think differently. We try to suppress the experience of the present. Ideally, we would control, map out, the experience of the future. We will look at the consequences of this shortly, but first we will attempt to explain the actual reason for this need or craving for control.

Reasons for our craving for control

Where do this craving for control, and this difficulty in allowing and accepting feelings come from? It's hard to say. The fact that controlling our environment *is* often effective appears to play a role. We are used to that.

Another explanation might be that it lies in our genes. In the past, human beings, like animals, had two effective ways of dealing with threatening situations: *fight* or *flight*. If the danger was too great, say you found yourself standing face to face with a grizzly bear, the wise move could be to make yourself scarce. If the danger was manageable or in the absence of other options, we would automatically put up a fight. These patterns of response are probably still present in our system.

Characteristics of our culture and messages passed on to us by our parents also seem to be important. An example of a cultural characteristic is the fact that we allow relatively little time for mourning. We consider it normal for someone to be sad and upset for a couple of weeks, but then we expect it to be business as usual. Examples of parental messages that teach us to control ourselves are: 'it'll toughen you up', 'big boys don't cry', 'don't carry on like that', and so on.

David mentioned once that he hated saying goodbye as a child. He was a very sensitive boy who made friends easily. He remembers going on holiday with his parents when he was fifteen. He had soon met a nice friend there, and they had spent 3 weeks hanging around together. When the friend left, he 'couldn't control his tears'. His mother said: 'Come on David, you're nearly grown up now. Saying goodbye is part of life: you should be able to cope with it'.

And don't we all have trouble coping with other people's sadness? Our reflex is to come up with quick-fix solutions. Or to ask probing, analytical questions. Or to say 'You'll be all right' and 'It'll turn out fine'. How difficult it is 'just' to be there, to lend support and to give someone space to be sad or despairing. If you allow the emotion in someone else, it brings your own buried feelings to light.

The mind leads us to ask pointless questions that only worsen the pain. Do you recognize the following questions or thoughts?

➡ Why am I feeling this?
➡ Why should this happen to me?
➡ What have I done to deserve this?
➡ Why am I like this?
➡ I don't want to feel this way.
➡ I can't control it.
➡ Etc.

1

You may have some favourites of your own that you could add. By analogy with the 'struggle switch' (Harris 2007) we call these 'struggle questions', questions that drive us to wrestle with ourselves. But what we are actually doing is tilting at windmills. These are questions that can't be answered. And let's be honest: they are also questions that allow us to feel sorry for ourselves, to play the victim and wallow in self pity. 'Look at me, look how badly off I am' is the message. And do we not ask these questions mainly because (once again) we are not prepared to accept a variety of situations and feelings? These questions magnify our powerlessness and only prolong an unpleasant situation.

They trap us again in the downwards spiral of living half a life. Questions like these are a sign that we believe we are entitled to positive emotions and happiness, and think it is normal in life not to have any negative emotions or unhappiness. To find happiness, we try to avoid or suppress negative emotions. But the harder we try, the more we reinforce them.

What we saw in Week 2 also applies to our ineffective control strategies. They tend to intensify the pain, rather than reduce it.

Think back to the scenario of the party and the unwelcome guest. This week, you are going to explore again how you handle control in your life, and what the consequences are. Because control and avoidance come so naturally to us all, it is our belief that you will give up these strategies only if you are truly persuaded that they will not help you to live in the moment.

Six statements about control in your life

Choose 'a' or 'b' for each of these six pairs of statements:*

1a   I need to control my feelings in order to be successful in life.

1b   I don't need to control my feelings in order to be successful in life.

2a   The best way of dealing with negative thoughts and feelings is to analyse them and identify the cause, so you know how to get rid of them.

2b   The best way of dealing with negative thoughts and feelings is to accept and allow them.

3a   I can only do something important when I feel good and sure of myself.

3b   I can often do things that are important even when I'm feeling gloomy or insecure.

4a   Having negative thoughts and feelings means there's something wrong with me.

4b   Having negative thoughts and feelings means I'm normal.

5a   I am afraid of my strongest feelings.

5b   I'm not afraid of my feelings, no matter how strong they are.

* Based on Harris (2007).

6a   It's bad to feel nervous.

6b   It's OK to feel nervous.

How many times did you answer 'a'? .... times

The more you answered 'a', the more likely it is that you have felt a strong need up until now to control your inner world.

Examples and consequences of control

Look again at the top five forms of psychological pain from Week 1 and answer the following questions.

What solutions have you tried in order to control your psychological pain?

1

How long have you been trying these solutions?

What has this all cost you? Think about money, time, energy, things you haven't done. Think too about the effects on your work, relationships and health.

> (blank box)

When you've answered these questions, how does this make you feel?

> (blank box)

Maybe now you feel a bit despondent, or sad, or dejected. Maybe you're angry with the authors of this book for asking these questions and making you feel like this. All we ask is that you notice your emotions, without judging, and bear them for a moment. We will return to them soon.

Messages from the past

In the introduction, we discussed how most people learn to manage and control negative thoughts and emotions in their childhood or adolescence. What message or messages have your parents passed on to you? In general, how were negative emotions handled in your family when you were younger?

1

Can you remember a time in the past when you felt intensely insecure, sad, lonely, abandoned, afraid or vulnerable? How did you handle it at the time? What happened?

We ask these questions to help you realize that your tendency to avoid or control is entirely human. The aim is to make you aware of automatic thoughts. These messages feel familiar and trustworthy, but they were only the opinions of the people who raised you. Opinions are not reality. No doubt your parents and carers had the best of intentions, but it may now be important to revise these opinions because they no longer suit your path in life.

Diary of painful moments and thoughts

Once again, we'd like you to keep a diary over the coming week of the times when you were bothered by a negative emotion or feeling. From now on, also try to write down the thoughts you had. Write down your emotion or feeling first, followed by the time and the situation, and then the accompanying thoughts. Include your response (your behaviour) as well. Finally, try to pin down any thoughts you had afterwards, in response to your behaviour and its consequences. In any case, the crucial thing is to fill in the diary at the end of each day. If something important happens to you during the day, it's a good idea to make a note of it so you haven't forgotten it by the evening.

A couple of examples are given to start you off:

Monday

Situation	7.00 am. Lying in bed, the alarm goes off.
Thoughts (1)	'Damn, I have to go to work again'.
Emotion/feeling	Listless, gloomy.
Behaviour	Turned over, then had to hurry.
Thoughts afterwards (2)	'That was stupid of me. I can't even get out of bed without messing up.'

Tuesday

Situation	5.30 pm. At home, around dinner time.
Thoughts (1)	'Why should I cook just for one?'
Emotion/feeling	Lonely.
Behaviour	Went to café and ate chips.
Thoughts afterwards (2)	'I'll get fat doing that. Then I'll be *totally* unattractive.'

Now fill in some situations of your own:

1

Monday

Situation

Thoughts (1)

Emotion/feeling

Behaviour

Thoughts afterwards (2)

Tuesday

Situation

Thoughts (1)

Emotion/feeling

Behaviour

Thoughts afterwards (2)

Wednesday

Situation

Thoughts (1)

Emotion/feeling

Behaviour

Thoughts afterwards (2)

Thursday

Situation

Thoughts (1)

Emotion/feeling

:::

Behaviour

Thoughts afterwards (2)

Friday

Situation

Thoughts (1)

Emotion/feeling

Behaviour

Thoughts afterwards (2)

Saturday

Situation

Thoughts (1)

Emotion/feeling

Behaviour

Thoughts afterwards (2)

Sunday

Situation

Thoughts (1)

Emotion/feeling

Behaviour

Thoughts afterwards (2)

This is another awareness-raising exercise. It helps you to become aware of thoughts that you have, and the way that feelings, thoughts and behaviour influence each other.

At the end of the week, try to answer the following questions for yourself:

➠ Looking at your diary, is there anything you notice?
➠ Are there certain thoughts that occur more frequently?
➠ Do you recognize any evaluative thoughts or compelling thoughts?

1

Alex is a 50-year-old man who had a heart attack 2 years ago. At first, he worked hard on his recovery, and it was going well. His physiotherapist was impressed with what he had achieved, which gave him a feeling of control. 'I've done a good job, I won't let it get the better of me'.

But it's not going the way he wants. 'It's those annoying emotions all the time. I never used to be anxious, I could take on anything and wasn't afraid of anything or anyone'. Now he's constantly taken by surprise. A tight feeling in his chest. Is it another heart attack? The cardiologist has reassured him that it's just panic attacks. What nonsense, he thinks, that's enough of that childish carry-on.

At night he has trouble sleeping. Gradually he becomes grumpier and grumpier towards his wife and children. When he starts to make mistakes at work and a colleague remarks on his bad mood, he finally seeks help. This is a very difficult step for him to take. 'What a load of drivel'. But thanks to the sessions, he learns that fear and anxiety are normal feelings and part of life.

The heart attack had been a huge upset. He realized that

he hadn't dwelt on it for any length of time. From being a healthy, active man, he had suddenly found himself staring death in the face. By not fighting the fear any more, he was able to make space for the experience. He also changed a number of things in his life. In the past he'd worked extremely hard, status was very important to him. He took a step back at work, giving him more free time. As a result, he now has time for an old hobby: music. He says his life is now more meaningful. Those around him think he has softened.

Mindfulness exercise: alternating body scan and breathing

Last week you practised observing the breath. Give a short description of the things you experienced.

The body scan and observing the breath are basic mindfulness exercises. The body scan increases your awareness of what is going on in your body. By being present with attention, you create space for sensations in your body. Physical sensations and your breathing take place in the present moment, in the now, whereas thinking catapults you to and fro between past and future. By practising the body scan and following the breath, you anchor yourself in the now.

Because these exercises are so important, we suggest that you alternate the two meditations this week. One day, do the body scan; the next day, observe your breath. Set an alarm to go off after 15 to 20 minutes. If you still find the exercise difficult, you can set the alarm to go off sooner.

A number of common queries and observations are addressed below.

I find it difficult not to alter my breathing. Yoga classes/singing lessons/relaxation exercises/breath training have taught me to feel the breath more deeply in my abdomen.

In the meditation exercise 'observing the breath', you follow the breath as it happens. The breath is fine as it is. You don't need to do or change anything. The exercise is simply about developing attentiveness.

However, it *can* be hard to let go of previous exercises. Other exercises such as yoga or singing lessons have taught you how to change the breath, and this can sometimes be useful. You have two options. The first is to notice that you tend to control the breath, so that you can let go of this tendency as time goes on. The second option is to follow the breath in a different place, not where you would usually follow it. For example, feel the breath flowing in and out through your nose (cool air coming in, warmed air going out). This may make you less inclined to change it. People who have had problems with hyperventilating in the past may also find this nicer to start with.

I get restless when I have to sit still.

You may well do. Especially if you're used to being busy all the time, sitting still is hard. Be aware that you're doing something new. You're learning a new skill. How do *you* go about learning something new? Restlessness is a normal feeling that can surface from time to time. Try to notice where you feel it in your body, and keep your attention there. If you can do this, you may be able to deal with it.

Be curious about your impulse to *do* something. In a normal situation, you'd probably have tried something by now in order to shake it off. Channel-hopping in front of the TV, pacing up and down?

The same is true of boredom. Boredom can raise its head if you sit still for any length of time. So it's a normal feeling, something you can notice. Try to keep your attention on the boredom.

The last time I practised, I felt relaxed. I'm not managing to get that feeling back.

Try to approach each practice with an attitude of openness and curiosity and notice what crops up from moment to moment. One day it may be a pleasant feeling, the next you may be overwhelmed by sadness or anger. Whatever it is, let it come and try not to aim for anything.

Being present in the now, with friendly attention, helps you to develop awareness. These mindfulness exercises are about developing awareness of what is there at present, not about pursuing a pleasurable feeling. By developing awareness, you gain an understanding of ingrained patterns. In the long term, this creates space for making different choices.

I'm a very down-to-earth person. I find meditating a bit airy-fairy.

This is a common misconception. Meditating makes you more aware of the present moment. Most people are trapped in the past or the future. Thoughts carry them off to far-flung places and different times. Who is more airy-fairy? Someone who is in contact with the now? Or someone who is living on automatic pilot, who is physically there, but whose attention is elsewhere?

It is also important to find your own form of meditation in which you can develop attentiveness. You don't need much in order to meditate. Some people like to dress their meditation up with rituals such as burning incense or candles. But if that doesn't suit you, it's not necessary.

Sometimes people look to meditation as a way out, an escape

from day-to-day worries, a break from everyday life. The exercises in this book are intended to help you to be present in the now. You develop this skill by giving attention to and connecting with whatever presents itself.

> *Meditation will solve my problems. I've heard that many people have really pleasurable experiences through meditating. Now that's for me!*

Be wary of (unrealistic) expectations. Starting with that assumption means you are not setting out with an attitude of openness and curiosity. A grain of scepticism can't do any harm. Practise, and experience what you experience. The aim is to develop attentiveness. If you have a pleasant experience, you can notice that. If your experience is not so pleasant, notice that as well.

Some people actively pursue a pleasant experience during meditation (perhaps by visualizing something nice). This can sometimes work really well. But remember that pleasant experiences are always fleeting in nature. If you pursue them, you will often be disappointed. And then can you embrace your disappointment with attention? Or will you start to engage in struggling? Or stop meditating?

> *Mindfulness is a gimmick, it's become a craze.*

Yes, there *has* been a huge surge in interest in mindfulness. That's a good thing. As far as we are concerned, the more people who try to live with a sense of awareness, the better. The exercises can certainly be used as a clever trick to help create some space for a while. However, in our view, mindfulness is ultimately about changing attitudes to life, about living with more attention and gentleness. This also applies to living outside the context of the 'official' exercises. Later in this book we will provide you with a number of tips for applying mindfulness in day-to-day life. For example, being present with attention while holding a conversation, folding the laundry, meeting people, answering the phone, cooking, showering, etc.

1

Metaphor: tug of war

We are now nearing the end of the first part of the book. You may have become aware of the amount of time you devote to battling your negative thoughts and emotions. It is a battle you want to win at all costs. You can't be happy until the anxiety, dark thoughts, eternal doubts, chronic pain, feelings of exhaustion, etc. have gone from your life. Only then can you get around to what you actually want to do in life. Only then can you be happy. Think back again to everything you've tried in your endeavours to win that battle. How much effort and energy you invest in it every week. It is truly a battle of life and death.

It's a bit like being in a tug of war (Hayes et al. 1999). Your opponents are your different forms of psychological pain, all tugging hard on the rope. Between you and them is a yawning chasm. If you lose, you will be dragged into it, never to be seen again. You're fighting for your life. You can't give up, so you pull harder and harder. But your psychological pain pulls harder and harder too. You start to tire. You feel the strain in your arms and legs. How long can you keep it up? You are forced to take a step towards the chasm. What next?

Write down your associations.

Continue to page 67.

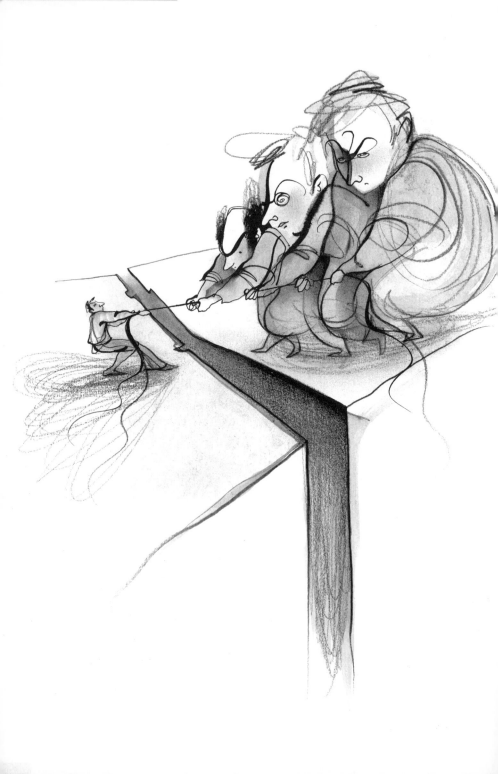

Stop and think

You have now completed the first part of *A Beginner's Guide to Mindfulness: Live in the Moment* and have gained a greater understanding of how you handle psychological pain and its attendant emotions. If you have realized that controlling and fighting that pain are not effective in helping you to lead a life that is more meaningful and worthwhile, you have already taken an important step. We hope you have a new found desire – or awareness of the need – to take action to give your life new direction and to let go of the familiar.

You will make a start on that next week. The next chapter is a key one on the path to a life worth living. The first step involves accepting negative emotions and being prepared to break out of the pattern of experiential avoidance. To that end, you will need to learn to leave your mind out of things, because the mind tends to give our inner world bad advice and to actually stand in the way of experience.

Experiences with learning

Take a look back over the past few weeks. How did you approach this book? Did you set aside time for it? What did you do if an exercise didn't work straight away? What were the most common thoughts that occurred to you? You should now be practising mindfulness on a regular basis.

Look back again at page 18. Do you recognize a recurring pattern with regard to learning in your life? Do you recognize your automatic responses? Being aware of them can help you to do things differently from now on.

➡ Are you someone who gives up quickly? Can you now give yourself more time?

➡ Are you someone who needs things to be perfect right away? Can you allow yourself space to develop?

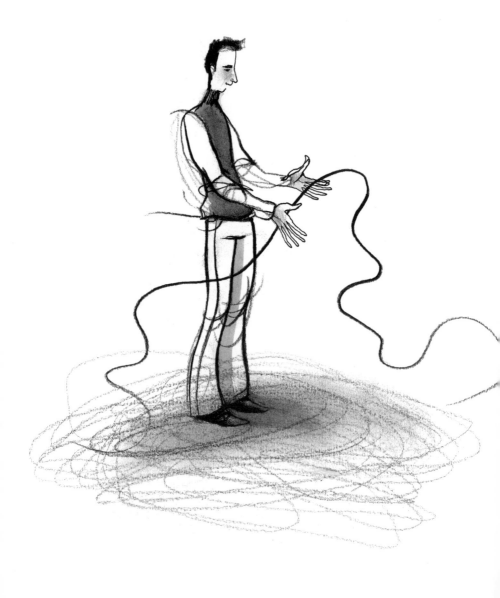

➡ Are you someone who seeks immediate results? Can you allow more time for the small steps?

➡ Do you have a tendency to race through the book without practising? Can you slow down, take time to understand, not only on an intellectual level but also on an emotional one?

Metaphor: tug of war (continued)

You can put down the rope!
You can decide to stop struggling.
You can let go!

Give this picture of a tug of war time to sink in. What did you feel at the end? Does it help you to realize how you have been approaching life up until now? Perhaps some other image comes to mind that represents your struggle with your inner world.

Confucius and the course of the water*

I follow the course of the water. . .
Sitting quietly,
doing nothing,
spring comes
and the grass grows by itself.
Zen proverb

One day, the philosopher Confucius and his disciples went on a trek to a waterfall with a huge, 150-metre drop. The foam drifted for miles and miles downstream. Not a turtle, fish or crocodile could get near the swirling mass. Then, to their

* A parable by Zhuangzi (also known as Chuang Tzu).

amazement, the company spied an old man swimming around in the churning water. He must be fighting for his life!

The philosopher commanded his disciples to save the man. But as they approached, he swam ashore, singing happily. His long hair hanging loose, he was enjoying the splendid surroundings.

Confucius went over to speak with him, and said: 'I took you for some sort of spirit, but now I can see you are a person. May I ask: do you perhaps have some special trick for swimming in this savage water?'

The man replied: 'No, I have no special skills. But I started to learn when I was very young, and as I grew up it became second nature to me. Now, a fortunate outcome is as certain as fate. I go with the current down to the middle of the vortex. I rise up with it again when it starts to turn the other way. I follow the course of the water without struggling against it. That is how I come through.'

Now return to page 63.

2

Resources for living in the moment

Week 4
Hello insecurity, welcome

When there is no way out,
there is still always a way through.
Eckhart Tolle

Introduction

Last week you learned that avoiding and controlling psychological pain doesn't work and in the end only worsens the pain. Your energy goes mainly into struggling with your pain, and that won't lead you along your chosen routes in the landscape of a life worth living. But what will? You have begun to realize that you're fighting a hopeless battle. The first and most important step you can take is acceptance. Acceptance is the readiness to feel what you are feeling at this moment, to experience what you are experiencing at this moment – even if your mind tells you it's better to run away, to suppress or diffuse the experience. It means being prepared to feel sadness, anxiety, insecurity, abandonment, anger, desperation, despondency, inferiority, etc.

Change is possible only on the basis of acceptance. This sounds paradoxical, but that's the way it is. Imagine you go for a walk in a vast area of natural beauty, and at some point you lose your way. There are a number of things you can do. You can lose your temper. You can give up. You can run off like crazy in a given direction. You can shout at the top of your voice. In many cases, these activities won't help. They're a waste of energy and you risk getting even more badly lost. Your confidence tumbles.

Your best chance of surviving is if you take stock of your

situation first; if you accept that you're lost. This also means accepting your feelings of uncertainty, loneliness and anxiety, but not giving in to the temptation of responding immediately to these emotions. Now you can try to orientate yourself, using all the tools you have at your disposal (map, position of the sun, features of your surroundings, visualizing your route so far). Then, you devise a plan that holds out the best chance of finding a village, a house or a path.

This example shows that acceptance is not the same as resignation (giving up, throwing in the towel). In that case, you allow yourself to be overwhelmed by the situation and the situation continues unchanged. That's the way it is in life as well. In order to bring about change where it is wanted (if we are not leading the life we'd like to live and are capable of living), we first have to accept and experience the situation as it is. All change is rooted in an awareness of the situation as it is. Without that, we are chasing dreams and fantasies, out of touch with reality.

Another reason why acceptance is so important is that life continues to flow. Impressions and experiences come and go. You can either go with the flow or struggle against it. Fighting it holds up the flow and stops you leading a satisfying life. You are trying to stem the flow of things you don't want, but things you do want are being held back in the process. Here is another example.

Imagine you're on a cycling holiday and the weather has been changeable, with sunshine alternating with showers all day long. Now imagine you decide you're not prepared to get wet today. What does that mean? For one thing, you will probably spend the whole day preoccupied with the weather. You'll be constantly peering at the sky, perched on the edge of your saddle. If you see another dark cloud approaching in the distance, you'll get off just to be on the safe side and go and seek shelter. Sometimes you'll be happy (if it does start to pour down 10 minutes later), but sometimes the cloud will simply pass by and leave you dry. If you follow this strategy, you won't get much out of the day or really be able to enjoy your surroundings and the cycling. The same applies if you start to peddle at top speed. Again, you won't enjoy your surroundings and the showers will probably catch up with you anyway.

Imagine now that you accept the inevitability of getting wet a few times that day. How does the day turn out then? You cycle more steadily and pay much more attention to and enjoy your surroundings. Sometimes you get wet, but the shower stops after a few minutes (the weather is changeable) and then you're even more pleased to see the sun. You feel the way the sun warms you and dries your clothes. You take the sun, rain and wind as they come, and will probably have a great day as a result. This is possible because you don't fight it. The rain is a nuisance from time to time but it never lasts long, it's only a passing thing. Your ability to experience the activity and your surroundings to the utmost is present all day long. At the end of the day you feel really contented. But if you fight the rain, you spend the whole day being obsessed with it! And in the meantime your enjoyment of the bike ride and your surroundings is impaired. You may reach that day's final goal, but you will probably be completely exhausted and won't have had a satisfying day that you experienced to the full.

Acceptance at various levels

As it is with the weather, so it is with our emotions and our psychological distress. If we accept these emotions, their influence is lessened, their duration shortened and we are able to live the life that we want to lead. But on the other hand, if we fight our psychological pain, we spend the whole day focusing on it ('anticipatory avoidance'), life comes to a standstill (we stay in our shelter on the off-chance it might start to rain), we waste our energy (by peddling madly in between the showers, which also dispels any holiday feeling, any sense of rest and relaxation we might have) and we are not doing what we'd like to be doing (enjoying ourselves).

Let's take a look at the effect it has on our lives when we refuse to accept psychological pain and negative emotions.

Paula has a drinks party to go to at work. She always feels tense in social situations and thinks it stupid and immature of herself to be so insecure. She'd rather not go, but today she decides to give it another shot. Walking through the room, she sees other people having a good time. She feels her own tension, the sweat trickling down her back, and rejects it: 'Here we go again, how stupid (evaluative thought), act your age, join in and enjoy yourself (compelling thought)'. Thoughts like these increase the tension without her realizing it. She starts to resist the insecurity even more, which only creates more tension. When a colleague speaks to her, panic gains the upper hand and she bolts, mumbling an excuse. Back at home, she feels like a failure and worries about how she came across to her colleague. (See the path of resistance in the diagram.)

2

The above example shows how clean pain (insecurity) leads, via evaluative and compelling thoughts, to dirty pain (increasing tension, panic). What would happen if Paula were to accept her insecurity? Insecurity is just something we have to deal with. The scenario might pan out as follows: Paula knows she feels insecure in social situations. It's an annoying feeling, but just one of those things. She can acknowledge its existence. If she observes it in a friendly way – 'OK, I am feeling insecure and here I am at the drinks party' – and then stays in touch with her feeling of insecurity without rejecting it, the tension won't mount and she will be able to stay. At the end, she'll be able to take pleasure in the fact that she put herself in a social situation. Even though it was hard (short term: clean pain), this will give her confidence that she'll be able to do it again the next time (see the path of readiness in the diagram.)

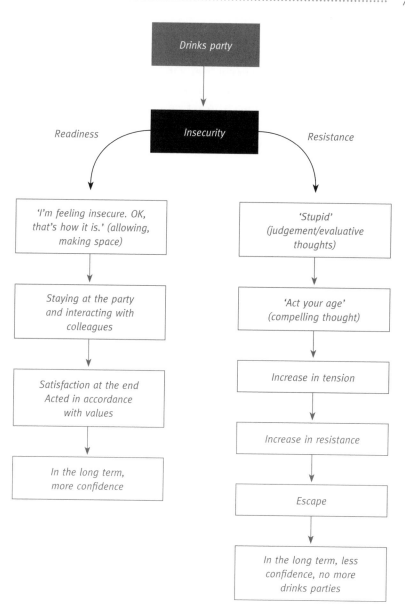

Readiness

The most important question we need to ask ourselves in order to break out of the impasse in our lives and head towards a life worth living is: am I ready to experience negative emotions and psychological pain? Am I ready to get wet? And in Paula's example: am I ready to feel insecure in social situations? There are other questions you can ask yourself:

- Am I ready to feel afraid?
- Am I ready to feel lonely?
- Am I ready to feel insecure?
- Am I ready to feel hopeless?
- Am I ready to feel gloomy?
- Am I ready to feel panicky?
- Am I ready to feel worthless?
- Am I ready to feel a failure?
  Etc.

and:

- So am I ready to put myself in situations that cause these feelings?

When you are fully ready to do these things, you can stop fighting or running away. You can stop your day-to-day struggles. You can let go of the rope that binds you to your pain. There is no room for compromise. You can only live in the moment, live a meaningful life, if you can say a whole-hearted 'yes' to painful emotions.

There are two ways to go about this. The first is by observing and staying in touch with your emotions. The second is by actually putting yourself in situations that will cause them. This week, you will undertake exercises doing both. We don't expect you to seek out the most difficult situations right away. You can work up to that step by step over time. And you will get support. You will learn about new ways of dealing with the thoughts that try to tempt you into rejecting experience. Moreover, you will learn that you are more than the sum of your thoughts, emotions and behaviour, so you will become kinder to yourself. But the effectiveness of this self-help book depends on your readiness to experience psychological pain.

What acceptance and readiness are not

Finally, we would also like to talk about what acceptance and readiness are *not*. First of all, as discussed above, acceptance is not the same as resignation. Acceptance does not mean passively having to accept life the way it is. That would mean that you are wholly a victim of your circumstances and that your actions wouldn't matter. Acceptance is an active, positive *embracing* of life. It is a way of saying 'yes' to life as a whole. The art is to strike a balance between acceptance and change. This is beautifully expressed in a saying ascribed to the seventeenth-century nun Teresa of Avila:

> *Give me*
> *the strength to change the things that I can.*
> *The courage to accept the things that I can not.*
> *And the wisdom to tell the difference.*

Second, acceptance is not the same as enjoying your pain. We do not invite you to enjoy your pain, to enjoy your psychological distress. That would be a form of masochism. You don't need to be happy with the distress in your life. Rather, we ask you to make friends with it, to familiarize yourself with it as part of your life.

And as for readiness, it is not the same thing as trying. This is the hardest and most important 'lesson'. When asked if you are ready to accept psychological distress, you can't answer with 'maybe' or 'I'll give it a try'. Half ready is not ready at all. When you say you'll give it a go, you actually mean you're not ready yet.

We are still in the realms of YES, BUT. There is still a little voice in your head saying 'if'. You are signing a contract, but it has an escape clause. 'If that situation arises, I'm out of here', is what you are saying. Readiness has only two options: yes or no. Nor does readiness mean maybe, tomorrow, next week, next year. Readiness is 100% now. When you say 'maybe', you're actually saying you're not ready yet.

So there is no room for compromise with readiness either. You may be saying 'yes', but meanwhile you're thinking 'no' or 'I'll see'. Or you secretly hope that being ready will bring you control of your feelings and experiences. But that is precisely what readiness will not bring you, and what it is not. You have a hidden agenda, and are actually still saying yes to only half of your life.

If you have doubts or find yourself haggling, it is a good idea to take time to allow everything you have read and learnt so far to sink in. Perhaps you're not yet convinced and want to try it another way first.

Be aware that, when you are ready, it is completely irrelevant how much pain you are experiencing! Readiness means that the focus is now on the content of your *life,* not the content of your *pain*. After all, you are setting your sights on leading a meaningful life, on being the person you want to be. That becomes the guiding principle, and the amount of pain becomes irrelevant! You have stopped battling your emotions.

Hayes (2005) gives the following definitions of readiness:

> Holding your pain as you would hold a delicate flower.
> Embracing your pain as you would embrace a crying child.
> Staying with your pain as you would stay with an invalid.
> Looking at your pain as you would look at an incredible painting.
> Doing justice to your pain as you would do justice to a friend by listening.

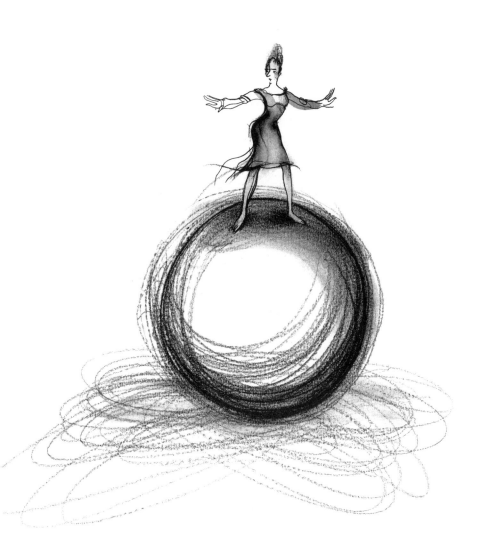

> Inhaling your pain as you would take a deep breath.
> Giving up your battle with pain like a soldier who lays down arms and goes home.
> Carrying your pain with you as you would carry a photo in your wallet.

There is also a beautiful poem that is cited frequently in mindfulness literature. It is by the famous Sufi poet Rumi.

THE GUEST HOUSE

This being human is a guest house.
Every morning a new arrival.

A joy, a depression, a meanness,
some momentary awareness comes
as an unexpected visitor.

Welcome and entertain them all!
Even if they are a crowd of sorrows,
who violently sweep your house

empty of its furniture,
still, treat each guest honorably.
He may be clearing you out

for some new delight.
The dark thought, the shame, the malice.
meet them at the door laughing and invite them in.

Be grateful for whatever comes.
because each has been sent
as a guide from beyond.

(translation by Coleman Barks 2004, reprinted with permission)

Why are you ready?

You have probably thought about whether you are ready to experience psychological pain in your life. We now ask you, in your own words, to give three reasons why you are ready to do so.

I am fully ready to experience psychological pain because:

```
................................................................

................................................................

................................................................
```

In Week 1 we gave the example of Iris, a woman who has been suffering from panic attacks since her father died. She had been working to conquer her anxiety for the past 8 years. She had tried everything and had become despondent. The book taught her that her battle was leading her even further away from her values (having new experiences, meeting people). She was able to recognize that her quest to overcome her anxiety hadn't helped. Previous treatment *had* given her some tools to use in the form of relaxation exercises, and she knew that avoidance didn't work. She had tried to control the anxiety. At the merest hint of it, she had started to struggle with herself. The resulting despondency began to tear her apart. Now she realized that she also had the option of accepting the anxiety. As she worked through the book, the travel brochure arrived in the post again. Am I ready to feel afraid? So could I actually make that trip in the long run? Am I ready to put myself in situations that cause me anxiety? Am I ready to allow this unpleasant feeling and take steps towards my values? The travel brochure helped her to make a decision.

Symbol of your distress: your bunch of keys

For this exercise (Hayes et al. 1999), we ask you to take your bunch of keys and lay them down in front of you. Choose two keys that you use a lot, e.g. your front door key and the key to the shed. Now imagine that these keys represent the top two 'sorrows' on your list from Week 1; the emotions you were fighting or trying to avoid. The front door key might represent your anxiety and the other key your insecurity. Now we ask you the following question: what are you going to do with these keys?

2

Continue to page 90 when you have given an answer.

Give your distress a name

Imagine you could sail to an island where there was no pain or distress any more. That sounds tempting: only contentment, youth, happiness, etc. from now on. It's a place where anything is possible. If you take time to get to grips with this idea, you will probably realize that it would dull your experience after a while. In the end you won't be happy with anything any more because you'll take it all for granted; you'll become lazier and lazier, you'll stop 'growing'. Life will soon begin to pall.

It sounds crazy, but the art of living is to welcome not only positive thoughts and emotions into your life, but psychological distress as well. Not because you're all that keen on distress, but because it is part of life and is also linked to understanding and growth; because distress (clean pain) means you take nothing for granted.

The following exercise is about accepting and dealing with psychological pain. Choose two of your thoughts or emotions that are currently giving you the most trouble. Give these thoughts or emotions a name. For example:

> Uncle Killjoy
> Auntie Can't
> Mr Critical
> Mrs Indecisive

Write down the names you have chosen.

Now, in the coming days, when you notice that thought or emotion creeping in, we ask you to welcome it by its pet name. For example:

> Ah, Mrs Self-Critic, so you're back again?
> Hi there, Uncle Killjoy, come on in.
> Hello insecurity, welcome.

Mindfulness exercise: making space and allowing what is there*

Read the following through carefully first, then practise every day.

We tend to have an aversion to 'negative' feelings (sadness, anger, fear, stress) and physical discomfort (an itch, pain). You have learnt that fighting these feelings only leads to more discomfort. It is impossible always to feel happy and contented and to go through life without pain.

The following exercise teaches you to make space for discomfort and pain. By giving them space, you may be able to diffuse these experiences. If you aim for 'if I just do my best, it'll go away', it won't work. You can do the exercise when facing negative feelings or pain, or you can recall a recent situation that you have not processed yet. In this case, the painful feelings associated with it will usually come to mind quite easily.

The exercise involves repeating a number of steps. Allow yourself time for the exercise. Make sure (especially at the start) that you are in pleasant, familiar surroundings.

1   Bring to mind a situation where you felt sad, angry or stressed.
2   Observe what is there at this moment. Note where you perceive this in your body.
3   Embrace this feeling in your body with your attention. Notice what happens. Stay open and be curious. Try to be gentle. Try

* Based on Kabat-Zinn (2001) and Segal, Williams and Teasdale (2002).

not to change anything. Allow what is there and what is happening.

4 After 5 to 7 seconds, observe what is happening: Is the feeling increasing? Changing? Staying the same? Is a different sensation coming to the fore? Notice where you feel this in your body. It may be the same feeling, or a different one.

5 Embrace this sensation with your attention. Even if nothing happens, embrace the unaltered feeling.

6 After 5 to 7 seconds, observe what is happening. Then go back to step 5.

7 Bring the exercise to an end after a while. If you like, you can revisualize the situation starting from step 1.

Bring the exercise to an end by following the breath with your attention for a while, as it happens from moment to moment.

The feeling may have changed, or maybe not. In any case, you have created space for the emotion or pain that you normally try to suppress. You may have discovered that you *can* bear these negative feelings after all. And that fighting them takes a lot of energy. If you *really* manage to accept the pain, you will notice that space has opened up between it and yourself. You will identify less with the pain. This space can have a liberating effect. However, it is very difficult for us not to pursue a goal. If you do this exercise with the aim of eliminating the negative feeling, you will find you have actually reverted to struggling.

Acceptance in action

It is important to take what you have learnt in this chapter and apply it in practice. In the box below, write down an action or activity that you have avoided recently. It should be an activity that does form part of a meaningful life. Choose an activity that can be carried out without too much preparation, and is not too difficult. It can be a challenge, but you needn't jump in at the deep end with the most difficult or exciting activity you can think of. Here are some examples:

> ❯ I'm going to talk to my partner about us spending more time together.
> ❯ I'm going to put my name down for volunteer work.

What is your activity going to be?

2

We would like you to carry out your activity in the next 2 days, and to allow any stress it causes you. If in doubt, think back over what you have learnt to date:

- ➠ Half a life is no life.
- ➠ I am reading this book because I want a meaningful, satisfying life.
- ➠ To that end, I will have to accept pain.
- ➠ If I try to avoid pain, it will only be worse in the long term.
- ➠ If you feel anxiety coming on, and an urge to pick up the rope and pull, you needn't give in to that urge!

➡ Keep your attention on the emotion, as you learnt to do in the mindfulness exercise.

Tip

You can also prepare for your activity by applying the mindfulness exercise 'making space and allowing what is there'. Visualize the activity and notice the accompanying sensations, embrace these with your attention. Every 7 seconds, observe what is happening. Repeat this a number of times.

Fill in below how it went.

Did you manage it? Congratulations. No, or not yet? That's a shame. Why not? Was it for practical reasons? Or did thoughts or emotions play a role? You can see this as a sign that you weren't quite ready yet to experience psychological pain. Practise again, using the mindfulness exercise for example. Attempt your activity again soon.

Metaphor: the struggle switch

As mentioned in the introduction, our minds can lead us to ask endless questions about a particular event. Something else we are good at is ANALYSING and looking for REASONS. We ponder endlessly over causes and how things came about. This doesn't actually get us very far; it only makes us feel more impotent. And it leads us to fixate on the explanations we have thought up.

ACT practitioners have devised an apt metaphor for this: the 'struggle switch' (Harris 2007). When we ask pointless questions, analyse, look for reasons or seek to apportion blame, we are turning on the struggle switch. Often, the result is that we start to get even more annoyed with ourselves.

When we do this, we are aggravating a second type of pain: indirect pain. As long as we are struggling, we are not devoting our energy to building a meaningful life. As a result, we are probably missing out on a number of positive experiences that we *would* have had if we had accepted the pain or negative experience sooner. If you find yourself asking pointless questions, analysing or seeking reasons in the coming weeks, try thinking of this image. It may help you to stop, or to laugh about it. But you can also see your struggling as a sign that you have not accepted the distress in your life and are not ready to make space for it!

2

Laura is a young woman who has her life fairly well-ordered. Health is a value that matters hugely to her. She plays sport and eats healthily. Her diary is pretty full: sometimes tiredness gets the better of her. She doesn't accept this but wonders why she is tired. And then she falls into a familiar train of thought that takes her back to an accident 10 years ago. 'Before that, I could tackle anything, now everything's different'. She thinks about what else has changed, and can recite a whole list. It makes her sad and angry. 'Why did this happen to me?' And then she gets furious again with the driver of the car that knocked her off her bike. Before she knows it, she is living it all again. Then she worries about the future. 'Is this going to continue? I'll never be able to function normally again'. This makes her anxious.

With the aid of mindfulness exercises, she learns to watch out for this ingrained pattern. She realizes that the questions she asks take her further away from her values, and the tiredness that triggered the pattern is still there. Her questions stem from resistance, and that doesn't solve the tiredness problem. Later, she learns what to do when she feels tired. For example, scheduling some space in her diary for doing nothing at all or simply lounging on the sofa. Thus, giving in to and making space for this feeling.

Tip

In the coming week, try to notice when you turn on the struggle switch. What effect does it have on you? Is it true that the struggle increases the more you fight it?

The art of living

In his book *De Vraag Naar het Lichaam*, philosopher Pieter Verduin discusses Nietzsche's philosophy of 'small' and 'great health'.

Small health equates health with well-being and purity. It is 'normal' not to be ill and not to suffer. Small health focuses on banishing distress. You might call it 'cosmetic psychology'. Everything is focused on making life pleasant. Small health invites us to commiserate with and feel pity for those who don't appear to be succeeding in this respect.

Great health embraces life in all of its fickleness, transience and ambiguity. It accepts distress and finiteness as ingredients of life. By refraining from fighting against distress and saying yes to a full life, we make space for the creative power of life itself. The art of living is the ability to celebrate life and to experience distress, to connect with specific ideals and to throw all of your talents into the fray. Great health invites us to feel empathy and solidarity.

Bunch of keys exercise (continued)

Did you pick up your keys? Congratulations! This shows that you are now ready to carry anxiety and uncertainty (or your chosen emotions) around with you and to allow them in your day-to-day life.

Did you leave them where they were? Or did you quickly stash them or throw them away? Consider for a moment what this means. First, you will find you keep coming back to check you've really left them there; so you can't go anywhere. And second, it is hard to live without keys; without them, you can't open some important doors. Is that worth it?

Now return to page 82.

2

Week 5
The 'trial balloons' of the mind

Our thoughts come in like waves
When they are there, they seem all the reality,
Total and forever.
The next moment they are gone and we just forget.
We are already busy with the next wave.
Jon Kabat-Zinn

Introduction

It happened again last night. At 3 am I jolted awake and immediately my mind started its incessant chatter. All the projects and activities I have to do went rushing though my brain. How am I going to work out such and such a problem? Is Joe angry with me, how did that chat really go? I'll never make that deadline and I've got an appraisal in 2 weeks' time. And I promised my father I'd help him pick out a new computer.

It was back again: the unstoppable 'train of thought' (Hayes 2005) thundering through my bedroom. This happens from time to time, usually when I have a lot on my plate. And each train compartment is crammed with night monsters: not a sheep to be seen. In my mind I've been sacked 50 times, fallen out with everyone I know, been divorced umpteen times, and the whole world knows that I'm good for nothing. In the dead of night I know all this with absolute certainty: that's the way it is. It's the inter-city night train hurtling past with its usual freight of alarming thoughts, sudden brainwaves and disaster scenarios. I've learnt not to let it get to me any more. 'Hey there, mind', I say to it, 'back to bother me again with all your worries and ideas?'.

The next morning, the world looks completely different again. All of those worries and disasters – and unfortunately the brilliant ideas as well – suddenly turn out to be not so worrying, disastrous or brilliant after all. And sometimes the night *has* brought me some good ideas: I really do need to revisit that chat with Joe; I could tackle that problem in such-and-such a way, it'll save me a lot of work. And I've noticed that if I welcome and observe the train of thought calmly, without getting worked up, it departs a bit sooner from the station of my mind. The *chug, chug, chug* fades away and I can catch a few more hours' sleep.

The train of thought shows up not only at night, but also in the daytime and at the most inconvenient moments. Our minds are constantly generating thoughts and playing us a wonderful, tragic film show of images. And those thoughts and images go round and round on an endless loop. If our boss asks to see us urgently: what have I done wrong? I must be performing below par! If we're on holiday abroad and someone rings us up: what's wrong? Who's died? I've left the gas on and the house has burnt down! And already we're picturing the house in a charred heap of ashes.

The mind produces thoughts and images as if on a conveyor belt. And it seems to have a marked preference for tragic, ill-fated, disheartening or upsetting scenarios. These thoughts and images can really put us off our stroke, so much so that there are times when we wish we could unscrew our heads from our bodies. Finally, a moment's peace. The mind seems to have a strong preference for fight and flight behaviour. It seems to encourage experiential avoidance: behaviour that we now realize doesn't help in achieving our goal of a meaningful and satisfying life. We can't 'unscrew' our heads.

Are there other ways of dealing with the mind so that it doesn't bother us so much? So that it becomes an ally who encourages us on our path towards a meaningful life, rather than an enemy who simply digs traps and holds up banners bearing

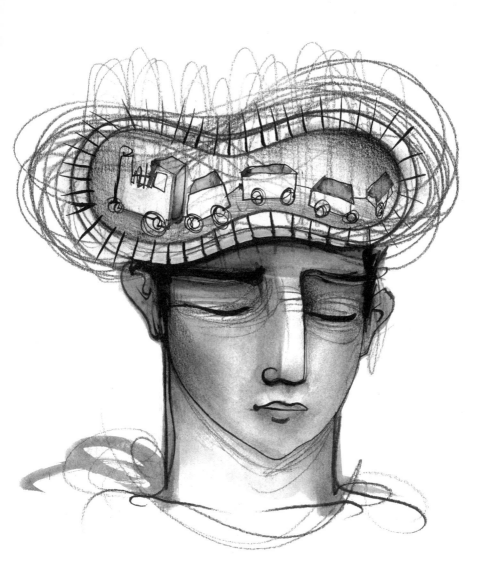

messages such as 'You can't do it, just give up' or 'Just go back to your pill-popping, drinking, eating or control freakery, at least you'll be rid of those nasty feelings'. We have good news for you. This approach exists, and it is called 'cognitive defusion'. And there's more good news. Anyone can learn cognitive defusion, it's free and it's fun into the bargain. But it does take daily practice.

What exactly are thoughts?

Let's start by exploring what thoughts actually are. Thoughts are words in our minds. And the formidable thing about them is that those words can be just as powerful as reality itself.

Imagine the temperature is a sweltering 35°C. You have a terrible thirst but there's no water nearby. Everyone will have experienced this. Are you there? Do you feel the thirst? While you keep reading, I go to the tap and fill a tall glass with water. Then I go to the fridge and open the freezer compartment. I feel the mist cooling my skin. I take out three ice cubes and put them in my glass. I take another ice cube and run it over my face, neck and throat, relaxing as I do so. Then I raise my glass of iced water and take a couple of deep gulps. I feel the cold water flowing into my mouth; how delicious water can be! I feel it running down my throat. A pleasant sensation runs through my body. I breathe a deep sigh and continue writing.

What happened to you? We'd be willing to bet, at the very least, that you became acutely aware of your mouth and palate and had to swallow. But isn't that peculiar? Because you were only reading words. Clearly, a few simple words are capable of becoming reality in your mind. Thoughts are words in the mind that can cause actual, physical sensations and emotions. Obviously, we can identify so closely with those thoughts in our mind that we mistake them for real, that they become reality. This is called 'cognitive fusion': automatically assuming our thoughts to be real.

This ability is also a source of great pleasure. Thanks to the power of the mind, words can appeal to our imagination so much that we lose ourselves in them. Take a book or a film for example. We can get so absorbed in the story that we forget ourselves and become one of the characters. We feel the same sensations: we share their highs and lows. Tears may even trickle down our cheeks, and at the end we are loathe to say goodbye. They may be only words and images, but for a moment they become 'all the reality'. The mind is a wonderful story-teller (Harris 2007).

But as is so often the case, this ability also causes us a lot of trouble. At the most inconvenient moments, the mind supplies thoughts and images that we experience as real and true, that undermine us and give all sorts of bad advice: You fool! What an idiot you are. You'll see, you can't do it. Precisely when they're not wanted, all sorts of thoughts crop up to make us feel ashamed and insecure. The difference is that we don't say them out loud. The mind can tell enticing stories. Take the tale of Odysseus for example.

Odysseus was an ancient Greek hero who wanted to go home after helping his people wage war against the Trojans. In the end, he succeeded but only after many ordeals and long detours. In one of his trials, Odysseus had to sail his ship past an island that was home to the Sirens, mythical creatures who sang so beautifully that no one could resist the temptation to land. But once you had gone ashore, you could never leave! Odysseus wanted to hear them sing so he ordered his men to tie him to the mast, while the crew put wax in their ears.

In this way, the mind can try to tempt us into experiential avoidance: just sit tight at home, at least nothing can happen to you there; you're still so tired, you can't go back to work yet; don't go to the gym today, your heart can't take it; if you finish the bottle, the pain will be numbed; just take those pills and you'll put an end to all the misery.

Sometimes, as Harris (2007) has it, the mind tells tales of deceit. It tells stories that would have you believe you're actually totally incompetent. If someone compliments you on your work, you don't accept the compliment because deep down you believe you're no good at anything. Soon you'll be messing everything up and it will become clear to all and sundry that you're only faking and you are actually having everyone on. You probably have a tale or two from your own experience that you can recount.

Cognitive defusion

The mind is therefore a great teller of stories. These can be stories that inspire us, encourage us, give us pleasure: stories that we are pleased to hear, and that we cherish. Unfortunately, they can also be stories – and, again, the mind seems to display a particular preference – that bother and undermine us. Ideally, we'd like to be less troubled by the latter variety!

In the field of ACT, a number of techniques have been developed in this regard. They reduce the power of these thoughts and help you to identify less with them. You begin to realize that a thought is only a thought, a story; it is not reality! Hence the term cognitive defusion. Fusion means merging or coming together, so by analogy defusion means easing away or separating.

You might want to try the following exercise, at night or in the daytime, either is fine! Take a thought that bothers you a lot. For example: 'I'm useless, I'm bound to mess this up'. Repeat this sentence a few times and try to really believe it. Then do the following. Keep saying: 'I have the thought that I'm useless, I have the thought that I'm going to mess this up'. What happens? Do you notice that the thought is already 'hitting home' a bit less, becoming less true? Every time your mind starts chattering away and generating annoying thoughts, say: 'I have the thought that. . ., I have the thought that. . .' You will find that, in a way, you are creating space between yourself and your thoughts.

This week you are going to practise a number of different cognitive defusion techniques. Your first task is to try them out and find out which of them works well for you. Then the crucial thing is to apply them frequently and consistently.

Defusion exercise 1

Write down five thoughts that bother you a lot.

Read these thoughts out loud and take careful note of what you experience.

Read these thoughts out loud again, but this time start each one with: 'I have the thought that. . .' Write down what you experience.

2

Continue to page 104.

Defusion exercise 2

Other defusion exercises (Hayes et al. 1999) that often work well involve saying the thoughts out loud and in a 'strange' way. In the coming week, practise the following options out loud every evening. Use the list from Exercise 1 and, if you like, add other thoughts that might be giving you particular trouble at the time.

⇢ *Say a thought very slowly.* Draw out each syllable of the sentence.

⇢ *Say a thought in a different voice.* Choose the voice of a film star, a cartoon character or another well-known person with a striking voice. Say your thought using that voice.

⇢ *A 'bad news' radio broadcast.* This one may work early in the day or if you have to do something that is causing you a lot of stress. For example, in an announcer's voice, say: 'At 1 pm today, Mr X will embark on an unusual venture, a task to which he is in fact completely unsuited. The whole country expects him to fail abysmally. More news to follow at 2 pm'.

⇢ *Exaggerating.* If you find you are judging yourself in a negative way, try passing extremely negative judgements on everything around you: what a miserable excuse for a door, call yourself a table, what a failure you are as a washing-up brush, who on earth created a doorknob like you, what an ugly lamp you are.

Write down your experiences.

Mindfulness exercise: observing your thinking

In the following exercise you become aware of the activity of your mind, namely thinking. Thinking is useful when dealing with practical problems. It helps us to analyse a problem and devise solutions. However, we also tend to use our thinking in situations where it doesn't in fact make any sense. In this case our thoughts influence us in a negative way. Thoughts can't be controlled. You *can* examine, after the event, if your thoughts were rational, but often this doesn't make them disappear.

This exercise teaches you to see what thoughts actually are. Thoughts are only events in your mind that come and go. And if you are preoccupied with the content of the thought, this will have repercussions for you. This is something else that the following exercise teaches you.

2

1   As in the previous mindfulness exercises, set an alarm to go off. Anything from 1 minute to an hour is fine.
2   Sit down in your usual position. Notice first how you are sitting on the chair, where your body is in contact with the chair. Then bring your attention to your breathing. Follow it for a number of breaths.
3   In the previous exercises, thoughts were still seen as a distraction from your meditation object (body or breath). In this exercise, it is your thoughts that are the object of the meditation. When thoughts come to you, notice that you are thinking.
4   If you like, you can label your thoughts. Identify what kind of thoughts they are: planning, judging, ruminating, worrying, analysing, remembering, chaotic (an interwoven mass of different thoughts) and so on. But don't force this naming process.
5   If this doesn't work, just be aware that thinking is going on.
6   Try not to label thoughts that have already slipped by. It is about the thoughts that are passing through your awareness at

this moment. Imagine you are standing at a conveyor belt of thoughts passing by. What has passed, has passed. You needn't pay it any further attention. You needn't strive to put a name to everything. Be kind to yourself.

7 As long as the focus is on the thinking, you are aware of the thinking or the type of thoughts. It is normal to become preoccupied with the content of your thinking and perhaps to drift far away. If you notice this, you can put a name to it, such as 'being carried away' or 'being preoccupied'.

8 Don't label the content of your thinking. Don't label the things you are thinking about, such as your work or your relationship. It's about the process: the type of thoughts you are having, or the fact that thoughts come and go.

9 It is not a bad thing to be carried away by your thoughts. By noticing this, you are developing your awareness of automatic patterns of thinking. Everyone has certain ingrained patterns that are triggered over and over again.

10 If there is an interval between thoughts, bring your attention to the breath. As soon as another thought comes along, identify the fact that you are thinking and, if you like, label the type of thought.

Metaphor: the waterfall

Jon Kabat-Zinn uses another apt metaphor to describe the phenomenon known in ACT as cognitive defusion. The mind produces a constant stream, or waterfall, of thoughts. You have two choices. You can go and stand in the middle of the flow and let yourself be swept along by its content. You can also go and stand behind the waterfall, looking at it and feeling the power of the thoughts, but not being carried along with them. Try to call up this image when meditating on your thinking.

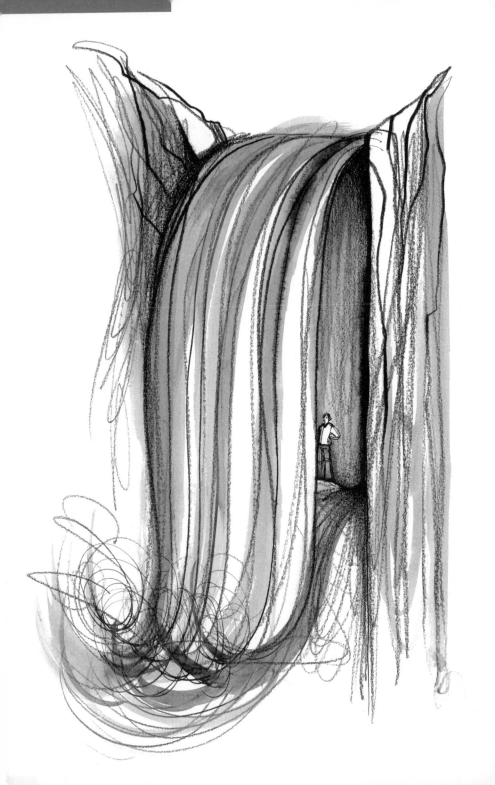

Metaphor: the landscape and the backpack

Imagine again that you are standing at the edge of the landscape of a meaningful life. You can see different routes through the landscape and the landmarks that will keep you heading in the right direction. You are carrying the backpack full of thoughts and stories. As long as you remain on the margins of the landscape, the contents stay relatively quiet and the backpack doesn't feel too heavy. But as soon as you start out on one of the paths towards a meaningful life, they begin to stir. They start to agitate, to weigh you down and try to pull you back towards the edge of the landscape. The thoughts and stories clamour more and more loudly: you will lose your way, a tree will fall on you, there's bad weather on the horizon, there's a grizzly bear on the path.

You have two options. Either you can turn back as they suggest, and the 'baggage' in your pack will settle down again. Or you can thank your mind for all of its useful trial balloons (stories and thoughts) but keep going in the direction that, to you, represents a meaningful life.

Over the coming week, try to call this image to mind when you are tempted to avoid or to start struggling with psychological pain.

FAQs and pitfalls

When should I, and when shouldn't I, apply cognitive defusion?

The mind will always generate a constant procession of thoughts and stories. That's its job. And don't forget that the mind is also a valuable ally that aids our survival. So thank your mind for the thoughts it generates. What your mind is actually doing is sending up a constant stream of trial balloons (thoughts, images, ideas). You can decide whether to pay them any attention (turn them into reality) or just let them be what they are: trial balloons. If you don't hold on to one, it will drift away or shrivel up by itself. Apply cognitive defusion when thoughts are not helping you to live a meaningful life.

Is the aim to eradicate these negative thoughts?
No, certainly not, and indeed that is impossible. The mind will always continue to produce negative thoughts. All we aim to do is to stop fighting our negative thoughts. Fighting them turns on the 'struggle switch' again! We resume the battle against our psychological distress and try to regain control. We pick up the rope again and start to tug, though we know that this battle is exhausting and that we can never win. Insecurity, doubt, sadness and pain are emotions caused by the thoughts and stories of the mind. They are part of life.

Does it matter if thoughts are real or not?
This is irrelevant in mindfulness and ACT. Both negative and positive thoughts come and go. It is about what you do, whether you are living according to your values – separate from the thoughts you have.

Cognitive defusion exercise 1 (continued)

You probably found the second time that your thoughts were becoming less true, less real. That is precisely what is meant by cognitive defusion. You create space between yourself and your thoughts. Try to apply this regularly in the course of this week. If you find yourself being plagued again by all sorts of troublesome thoughts, keep saying: 'I have the thought that. . .'.

Now return to page 98.

Week 6
Who exactly am I?

You can try to become free of problems.
You can also try to become free in your problems.
When you say 'yes' to the 'isness' of life,
when you accept this moment as it is,
you can feel a sense of spaciousness within you that is deeply
peaceful.
Eckhart Tolle

Introduction

This week is about attention. Specifically, the hardest kind of attention there is: loving attention for ourselves.

I often get up very early to take the train to work. Some days, when the sky is hazy and scattered with wispy clouds, I am treated to the most amazing sunrises. It strikes me too that these sunrises go unnoticed by most people, who are engrossed in conversation, buried in the newspaper or still lazing in bed. I feel an urge to shout 'people, look at this, pay attention to the dawn for a moment!' So far, I've managed to suppress that urge. Some days, in any case, I'm probably absorbed in a book myself and the person sitting across the way is thinking the same about me.

So many moments pass by in which we are busy with something (in our heads, in our future or our past) and fail to pay attention to what is actually happening to us in the here and now. Even though attention is a vital precondition for leading a meaningful and fulfilled life. Let us explain what we mean.

The value of attention

Attention is the ability to notice what is happening to us in the present moment. Attention is attentiveness, or 'mindfulness'. It means observing, but not just that: it means being fully present in the moment. We are experiencing the situation. We are aware of what is going on. Attention is perhaps our most precious possession. What is love, if it is not first and foremost being there for someone, being present, listening? What is friendship, if it is not knowing that someone is there (giving you their attention) when you need them? Is attention not the most important condition for growth? Is loving attention not the opposite of emotional neglect? Attention is a scarce resource. You can't give your attention to everyone and everything at once; you can only focus on one person or one activity at a time. That's what makes it so special.

Living with attention is the opposite of living on automatic pilot, something else that we have all experienced. Eating a meal, but not actually tasting your food. Reading a book, but not taking it in. Going for a walk, but not noticing your surroundings, the scent of the wood or trees. Physically, we are there but our minds are elsewhere so we are not truly experiencing.

Living with attention is also the opposite of living unconsciously. We do a huge variety of activities, and ideally as many as we can, but why do we actually do the things we do? Do we undertake a given activity (say visiting our mother in the care home) because it is expected, because we feel obliged or because we want people to think well of us? Or do we do things because we regard certain values as important, because we have made choices?

In the coming week we will see that living on the basis of an awareness of values and choices is much more satisfying, and you will spend some time thinking about the values that matter most to you.

But there is a second reason why attention is so important.

Without it, there is no possibility of change. In order to change something, we must first of all have noticed it. We need to pay attention to what is happening, what is going on. We can only change our behaviour if we notice everything that precedes it (environmental stimuli, physical sensations, thoughts, feelings). If you notice something, you have the option of deciding how to tackle it. If you go through life without noticing things, you are functioning on automatic pilot.

This is why we have devoted so much attention to mindfulness from Week 1. The ability to focus on what is happening to you here and now enhances the quality of your life and makes choices and change possible. This makes it a vital condition for a meaningful and satisfying life.

'Doing mode' and 'being mode'

There is yet another way of looking at attention and attentiveness (Segal et al. 2002). Human beings have two states of mental function: 'doing mode' and 'being mode'. Mindfulness is the ability to switch from doing mode to being mode. In being mode, you are fully in the now.

Being mode focuses on accepting and allowing what is there. Thoughts and feelings are noticed and observed as they occur. They are events that crop up, receive attention and disappear again. You can observe your thoughts and feelings in the same way as you might look at a river. You observe the leaves, twigs and other objects and let them gently drift by. 'Being mode' is a state of absorption in the now and hence timeless. It involves no judgement or evaluation, no right or wrong. The basic attitude is one of acknowledgement: *'it is as it is'*. I notice it and it passes by. There is no comparing or assessing.

Being mode has a soothing and broadening effect, creating room for movement. In any case, it gives rise to a greater ability to experience unpleasant emotions without automatically triggering unproductive response patterns.

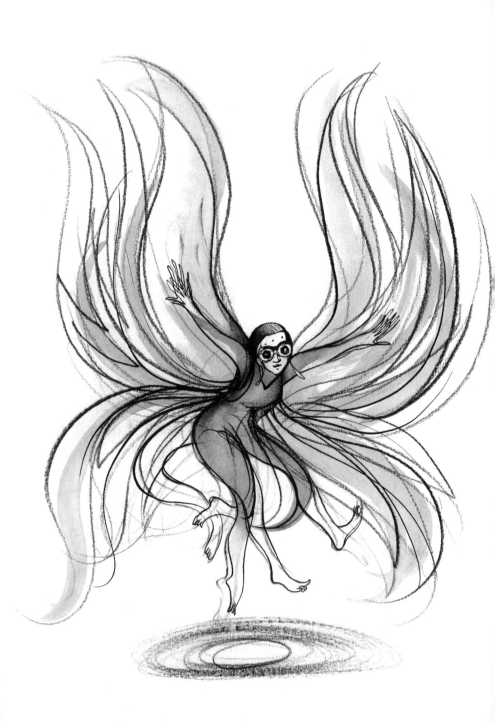

Doing mode is an action mode. Doing mode always kicks in on the basis of evaluation. You notice something that is undesirable, too much or too little, and you have an immediate urge to eliminate this discrepancy between an undesirable and a desirable situation. Something needs to be done, because it can't go on like this. This process is often automatic. A solution is needed, so the situation must be analysed and goals set. The most common feature is a feeling of dissatisfaction. There is a lack of acceptance. The basic attitude is one of *'it's not right as it is'*. Clearly, doing mode carries us away from the now. Doing mode is useful for external problems, but tends to lead to frustration and stagnation when dealing with internal problems.

When you experience and appreciate this difference, you will probably understand more why we said in the first chapter that half a life is no life. An immediate discrepancy arises. You end up literally under stress (in a state of tension), because things aren't right the way they are; this leads to a feeling of dissatisfaction. If you don't reach your goal, you feel even more unhappy. And if you do achieve your goal but can't achieve 'being mode', right away there is another new goal and hence a new discrepancy!

So are we asking you to stop doing things? To stop taking action, to stop making more plans? To stop taking new steps? Of course not: that is impossible and nor is it the intention. Life demands that we make decisions and live by them. The difference is in how those decisions are made: freely or on automatic pilot. Being mode allows you to make decisions with attention and awareness and based on your values, not because you feel compelled or from fear of censure. The art of living is to know when to accept and when to act.

Do you have the patience to wait
till your mud settles and the water is clear?
Can you remain unmoving
till the right action arises by itself?

Lao Tse (also known as Lao Tzu)

The observing self

Now, however, a crucial question arises. We have gradually come to the realization that we are not our bodies, but we are also not our thoughts. Who are we then? We are none other than the ability to experience every moment. Physical sensations, emotions, thoughts and impressions come and go all day long. But someone is constantly present, and that is your 'observing self'.

Now we have another question for you. That observing self, that part of you that is aware of what you are doing, feeling and thinking all day long, is it good or bad? Or is it 'just' present? There is only one possible answer, and it is the latter. The observing self can only observe and experience (it cannot think or feel), so it can't be good or bad. And the observing self can never judge or evaluate, because judgements and evaluations are thoughts, and the observing self cannot think. Nor can you improve the observing self, because it is constant.

Harris (2007) gives the following description of the observing self:

- The observing self is there from birth to death and is unchanging.
- It observes everything you do, but never judges you.
- It cannot be hurt or damaged in any way.
- It is not a 'thing'. It is not made of physical matter.
- It cannot be improved on in any way; therefore it is perfect.

These traits make it a permanent source of true acceptance. It is up to you and within your power to 'connect' with it. And that is good news! Because that puts us on the track of loving attention for ourselves.

If we were to ask you what Jesus, Buddha, Confucius and Gandhi (past and ongoing sources of inspiration for so many) have in common, what would your answer be? There are many potential answers, but gentleness and loving attention for everything there is are certainly among them. These spiritual leaders were not happy with everything, but their basic attitude was one of gentleness; they had a non-judging frame of mind. And isn't that the hardest thing to put into practice? Not being too quick to judge and condemn other people? But particularly ourselves. After all, we are masters of self-criticism and find it extremely hard to be loving towards ourselves.

Lazy, boring, stupid, selfish, dull, predictable, a failure, ugly, too fat, shy, etc. how readily we slap such labels on ourselves. And isn't 'lack of self-confidence' the totemic phrase of our times, the one everyone uses to explain why they're not doing what they'd like to be doing? 'I'd sign up for that course but I need more self-confidence first'. We are constantly labelling ourselves, telling discouraging tales about ourselves. We have all experienced to some extent how hard it is to change that; often we've already given in to the self-criticism. Because how on earth do you do that: how do you learn to love yourself more?

The answer is in the previous paragraphs. By connecting increasingly with your observing self, and staying in being mode more often, you develop a greater understanding and love for everything you observe and approach with attention. Presence makes the heart grow fonder! By observing when you are judging and condemning, you start to judge and condemn less. You become calmer and friendlier. Towards others, but also towards yourself.

Mindfulness exercise: anchoring

This exercise can help you to notice how things are with you at this moment. It also helps to anchor you in the here and now and to bring you into being mode. The exercise consists of three steps, each of which can take around a minute.

1   Notice what is to the forefront of your being at this moment.

Are there any thoughts, physical sensations, emotions, noises, smells or sights? Observe and acknowledge what is there at this moment. If you are sad, notice the sadness. If you are happy, notice the happiness. If there is a lot of noise, notice that you are hearing. If you find you're looking around you, notice your awareness of seeing. If you feel any pain, notice the pain. And so on.

2   Bring your attention to your breathing. Try not to direct or control the breath. Your breathing is fine as it is. Follow it for a number of breaths.

3   Now expand your attention to your body as a whole, including your breathing. You don't need to scan every part of the body. Embrace your whole body with your attention.

This exercise can be practised frequently in the course of a day. Spare moments are ideal, moments when you have the time and space to develop attentiveness. For example, you might practise while waiting to see the doctor, waiting for a train, bus or for your computer to boot up, as you sit at a red traffic light, or simply when you manage to clear a space.

Judging exercise

There are two ways of looking at ourselves and the world around us: from the perspectives of the 'observing self' and the 'thinking self'. From the perspective of the observing self, we mainly perceive the form, without judging or evaluating. This takes us into being mode more quickly. The thinking self focuses more on content: we analyse, judge and evaluate. This takes us more easily into doing mode. It is useful to develop the skill of noticing when you are seeing the world from these two different perspectives. One way to practise this is by consciously changing your perspective.

Here are some examples.

Observing self	Thinking self
It's raining.	The weather's bad today.
Harrison Ford is an actor. Harrison Ford appears mainly in action films.	Harrison Ford can only play one role: himself. Harrison Ford is a brilliant actor.
I feel like working late this evening.	If I don't work late this evening, I won't get finished and the consequences will be unpleasant.
I have the judgement that I had an unhappy childhood.	I had an unhappy childhood.
I have the thought that Sundays are dull.	Sundays are often dull.
I feel like going for a drink.	I need a drink now or I'll lose it completely.
I notice anxiety.	I am a scaredy-cat. Anxiety is bad.

Do you see the differences? Now try to switch from one perspective to the other as you look around you, and try to notice what physical sensations you have in the different perspectives. For the first minute, identify what is happening within you and what you think about everything around you, and about yourself. For the second minute, identify only the facts and what you are doing. Switch perspective a few times.

Write down what you notice.

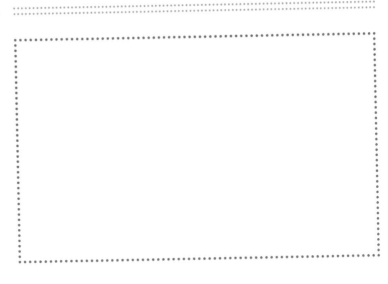

Comparing exercise

Comparing takes you even further away from what is happening now. Comparisons enhance or diminish your assessment of self-worth. Comparing usually entails a judgement: more than, better than, less than, worse than. Comparing is a typical 'ego activity'.

Comparing self

What wonderful scenery, but I found the scenery in France last year even more beautiful.

Her hair is much nicer than/not as nice as mine.

My neighbour is off on holiday again. He must earn a lot more than I do.

Why can't my kids be as studious as my brother's?

Comparing is often characterized by an inability to accept the situation. We ask you this week to record a couple of occasions when you find yourself comparing. Write down an example every day. Try to notice what you are doing, and when.

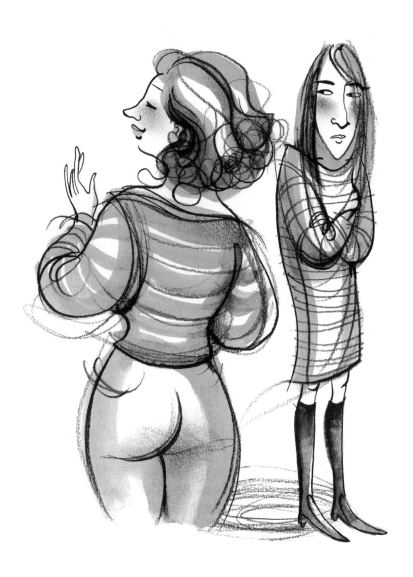

How often do you tend to compare?

Do you find comparing a satisfying activity?

2

What do you recognize as the themes (appearance, possessions, status, knowledge, performance, qualities, etc.) of your comparing?

Now read the text on page 121.

Photos and life story

We want you to select five photos, in which you appear, of situations from your life and to lay them on the table in front of you. The photos should be from different periods in your life. For example, someone in their 50s could choose a photo from their childhood, one from adolescence, one from around the age of 21, one from their 40s and a recent photo.

Look at the photos carefully and answer the following questions for each one:

⇒ Where are you?
⇒ What is the scene?
⇒ Who else is there?
⇒ What do you look like?
⇒ What is your mood?
⇒ What are you doing?
⇒ What are you focused on?

When you have done that, answer the following questions:

⇒ Who is the person in the photos, and who is the person looking at them now?
⇒ What are the differences?
⇒ What has stayed the same?

Photo 1

2

Photo 2

Photo 3

Photo 4

> *Photo 5*

Next, we want you to consider the different roles you play in your life. How do you behave in each role? And how do you experience each role? Roles may include the following:

> partner
> child
> brother or sister
> parent
> friend
> neighbour
> colleague.

In each of these different roles there will always be a part of yourself that is different. But is there also a part of you that is always the same? Describe that below.

Continue to page 122.

Tip: stay small

2

In his book *A New Earth* (2009), Eckhart Tolle writes about the art of staying small. This is a good exercise to do in order to stay with the observing self and to be kind to yourself. Sometimes you meet someone who makes you feel small in comparison. They talk about successes in their life, for example, and appear self-assured. Your automatic pilot response may be either to start feeling inferior or to respond with various success stories of your own, in order to feel 'bigger' again. If you find you are starting to feel small, try to allow this and stay loving towards yourself. You may just realize that you are fine the way you are.

Metaphor: the sky

The observing self could be said to be like the sky. The clouds are constantly changing. Sometimes it rains or thunders, and sometimes the sky is a brilliant blue. At night the moon comes out and the stars change their positions. But the sky always stays the same, itself.

Let this metaphor sink in for a moment. What do you notice?

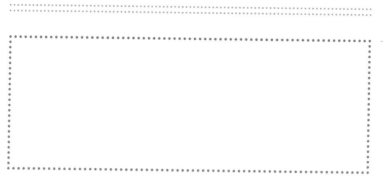

Comparing exercise (continued)

This exercise shows Anna that she does an awful lot of comparing. She compares her children's development (their motor skills, their vocabulary) with that of her brother's children, who are around the same age. At work too, she is constantly comparing herself with her colleagues: whether her hair is nicer than other people's, or not so nice, what everyone is wearing, etc. Sometimes she comes out on top, sometimes she doesn't. The main thing she finds is that it makes her agitated; she needs constant affirmation.

Constantly comparing is a typical activity of the thinking self. In a sense, you are always identifying with content and form. Your day-to-day self-esteem depends on things and people around you. One day it is sky high, the next it plummets. Comparing doesn't help you to live in the moment.

Living in the moment is done on the basis of essential motivation and values, irrespective of what other people think or do. If you do experience things in this way, there is a risk that you will start to condemn your comparing. That is not the intention. Mindfulness can help you with this. Try simply to notice your comparing, with compassion and with a smile. Then you will probably find that you need it less in the long run.

Now return to page 116.

Photos and life story exercise (continued)

You may have noticed the following. Your life (or way of living) has changed over the course of time, and a lot has happened in your life. You behave differently in the different roles you currently inhabit in life.

But is it not also the case that part of you was always there, is always there and will always be there? You are not your body, you are not the events in your life, you are not the thoughts and feelings that constantly come and go, you are not the behaviour that you display in different situations. You are the person who sees all of this, who was always there and always will be. You are the ability to observe and be aware.

Take a moment to explore how this realization affects you.

2

The ego

An author who writes a lot about mindfulness and the thinking and observing self is Eckhart Tolle. In *Practising the Power of Now,* he focuses on the importance of living in the now as far as possible and observing everything around us with maximum attention. In *A New Earth,* Tolle writes at length about a major obstacle to living in the moment: the ego. The ego is the part of us that becomes absorbed in thinking and doing, without attention or awareness. It is our automatic pilot. The ego is linked to the concept of self. This concept develops in children on the basis of identification with their own name, possessions (toys, mummy and daddy, etc.) and other things, and later with thoughts about those things. The ego therefore identifies with form and content – the thinking self – and always wants more. This makes comparing a typical 'ego activity'. The nicer our homes, the fitter our bodies and the more money we have in the bank, the more we are worth, reasons the ego, and it is always satisfied only in the short term.

Cognitive defusion, mindfulness and expanding the

observing self, accepting pain and living on the basis of values imply a smaller role for the ego. The ego wants you to stay put in your shelter, defending your possessions and not taking any risks. Complaining, bearing malice, comparing, judging and justifying itself are the ego's favourite pastimes. The ego forces us constantly to live half a life. It tries to tempt us to keep searching for that island without pain or distress. The ego puts us in doing mode. This doesn't mean that you can't enjoy a nice house or car, or take pride in your achievements. On the contrary. The important thing is not to base your self-esteem on these things automatically, to realize that the essence of who we are is completely separate from form. If you can start to feel that more intensely, and we hope this book will help you in that respect, you will become more stable, less hurried, more gentle. You will develop a keener eye for the things that connect people.

Now return to page 120.

Stop and think

You have now completed the second part of this book, and have practised the most important conditions for living in the moment.

If all has gone well, you are now able to notice negative emotions and thoughts and to stay in touch with them (not run away). Your mind doesn't carry you away so much: you have stopped automatically treating your thoughts as reality. Your mind has become a servant again, rather than a master. You have experienced what it is like to be in being mode and have become aware of your observing self.

These skills or arts of living do require constant practice. You will often fall back into old patterns. That is all part of the process. Something you've been used to doing for a long time cannot be unlearnt in a matter of weeks or months. What matters most is that you start to notice it (earlier and earlier in the long term) and that you are able to adjust. Your observing self assumes a bigger role in your life and your ego takes a step back. You start to move more with the flow (and counterflow) of life, rather than fighting or controlling it. This will ultimately give you flow in your life. You will have a keener awareness of what you do want in your life, and what you want to shed. In the next and final section, you will take this a stage further. By making choices in your life and committing to them, you will enable living in the moment to take stronger root and develop into a sturdy tree capable of withstanding all weathers.

STORY

2

*If a man is crossing a river
and an empty boat collides with his own skiff,
even though he be a bad-tempered man he will not become very angry.
But if he sees a man in the boat,
he will shout at him to steer clear.
If the shout is not heard, he will shout again,
and yet again, and begin cursing.*

*And all because there is somebody in the boat.
Yet if the boat were empty,
he would not be shouting, and not angry.*

*If you can empty your own boat crossing the river of the world,
no one will oppose you,
no one will seek to harm you.*

Zhuangzi (also known as Chuang Tzu)

3

*Living in
the moment
in practice*

Week 7
How do you want to live in the moment?

Some people achieve the top of the ladder
and only then realize it was standing against the wrong wall.
Stephen Covey

Introduction

Have you ever been cycling through some woods or meadows and suddenly come across a magnificent, distinctive tree? Strong, full of character, with a luxuriant canopy. A tree with personality. A tree that you look on in admiration and amazement. There are trees like this everywhere. Doesn't a tree make a good metaphor for a worthwhile, satisfying and meaningful life? Wouldn't you like to stand firm in life like such a tree?

Acceptance, cognitive defusion and mindfulness could be seen as the roots of the tree. They are its life lines, taking and transporting nourishment from the earth. But this depends on earth as a source of that nourishment. What nourishes a worthwhile and satisfying life? The answer is inspiration, which is contained in abundance in values. Without an awareness of values that matter to us, it is not easy to lead a worthwhile and inspired life. In this chapter we will look at the subject of values in more depth.

Trees have another important feature: they are steadfast and enduring. A worthwhile life does not develop overnight – it takes mental tenacity and commitment. It takes the drive to actually connect with those values, to give them a place in your life through choices and activities. Commitment is addressed in Week 8.

What do you want out of life?

We asked this question at the start of the book, mainly in order to make you aware that the obvious answer ('happiness, prosperity!') is not a good guiding principle and can in fact sustain an unhappy life. It tends to put you on the defensive (focused on control) rather than the offensive. We will ask the question again, but this time more potently, more forcefully. You can only achieve what you want to achieve – a worthwhile, satisfying and meaningful life – if you are pervaded by a strong sense of the values that matter to you. You want to live in the moment. We will now look at *how* you plan to do that.

Most of us only really become aware of what we want out of life when something bad happens, such as when a loved one dies, a serious accident befalls us or we learn that we don't have long to live. It's like a sudden wake-up call. We make life-changing decisions, and experience day-to-life life and relationships more intensely. Up until then, we were living mainly on automatic pilot.

But suppose nothing like that happens (and we don't wish it on anyone), are we prepared to reach the end of our lives only to find that we haven't lived every moment to the full? That we didn't engage enough with whatever it was that really mattered to us, that we didn't step forward and speak out enough, that we didn't take great pleasure in the extraordinary within the everyday? 'Life is short' is a cliché, but no less true for that. And, as everyone knows, life can come to an end without warning.

We now have two options. We can forget that life is finite, bury our heads in the sand and allow ourselves to be guided by the demons in our backpack; or we can make a start now by picturing ourselves as old men and women looking back over our lives and by imagining what we'd say to ourselves. We invite you to explore your personal values and to create a space for them in your life.

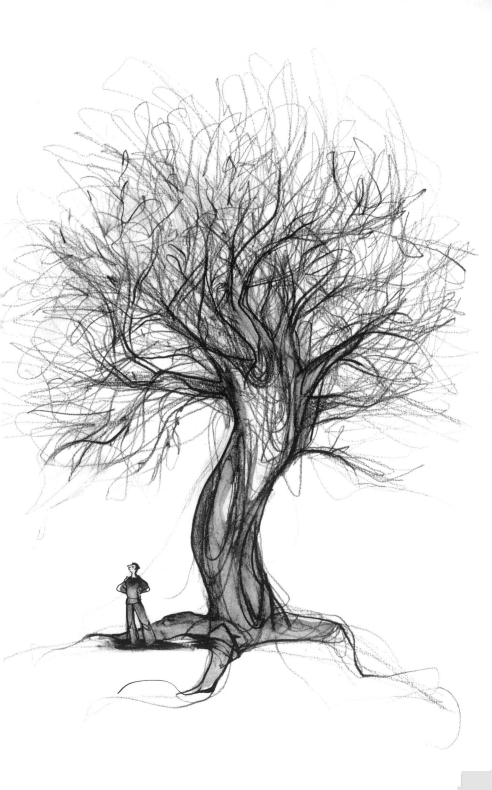

Steven Hayes, the founding father of ACT, defines values as 'chosen life directions'. Values point to the things that matter most to you in life, that make life worth living for you, that inspire you. Values are like the four points of the compass. They help you to determine your direction. This may become clearer if we explain what values are *not* (Hayes 2005).

3

➠ *Values are not goals.* This is important to realize. Goals are specific, achievable results. If your goal is to walk to a town, you may find at some point that you have reached that goal, perhaps when you see the 'Welcome to . . .' sign or when you reach the town centre. But if you have chosen to 'walk east', there is no finishing point. The only thing you can check is that you are heading in the right direction, that you're on course. In principle, there is no final destination.

➠ *Values are not feelings.* 'Enjoying yourself' or 'wanting to be free from pain' are not values. You either have, or don't have, a given feeling. You can 'possess' it. Not so with values. As soon as 'wanting to be free from pain' or 'enjoying yourself' becomes your guiding principle, you are seeking to control your life; it encourages you to live not a whole life, but half a life. And is 'enjoying yourself' really a source of inspiration for a satisfying life? Does it encourage you to take steps in your life that you find difficult but know are important? No. But values *do*.

➠ *Values exist separately of the result.* Doing is more important than the outcome. Imagine it is important to you to have affectionate contact with your mother, even though she ignores you. Because this value matters in your life, you send her a card with a brief message every month, say. Even if you never hear anything back, this can still continue to provide you with pleasure and meaning because you are connecting with your value. This often works the other way round as well. Imagine you are studying law because your father thinks it important and has put a lot of pressure on you. But you'd much rather be doing nursing because caring for people directly gives you a lot of satisfaction and is a value that matters to you. What happens when you pass your law exams? Will you experience personal satisfaction, deep contentment? Chances are you won't. As long as you are pursuing something that is not based on what really matters to you in life, it won't bring you deep satisfaction, even if you achieve it.

➠ *Values are not chosen by the mind.* The mind can think logically, analyse, make plans, etc., so we need the mind in order to achieve our goals. You consider what you need in order to achieve your goal and how to gauge if you are coming any closer to it. But goals are not values, as we discussed above, so the mind doesn't really come into it when dealing with values. Goals are useful as benchmarks, as aids to help you live on the basis of values. But first, you need to know what your values are. Values are chosen by the heart. You know you've got a value whenever you feel inspiration, whenever you find that something gives you energy and meaning.

Being in touch with your values makes you strong

The more deeply rooted a person is in his values, the stronger he stands. Think back to that distinctive tree. And the stronger you stand, the better you are able to support others. You can always apply values, even if life seems to be against you.

Living based on your values is not easy, especially at the start. Your own ambition, insecurity, or other personal traits can tempt you into setting too many goals that don't fit in with your values. Your mind will try to tell you, in myriad ways, that something is pointless or can't be done. You may live or work in an environment where everyone is constantly in doing mode.

Sometimes, living according to your values will lead you to make decisions that cause yourself or others pain or sadness, or fear of the consequences. In this case your mind may start to whisper that it's 'better not to', in order to spare yourself and the other person that distress. You will need to muster up strength to accept this and to apply cognitive defusion. But the vital thing is to stay in regular, day-to-day touch with your values. And that you do so by making regular contact with the 'being mode', by focusing on what is going on inside you and what is there now. And then, as Lao Tse (see page 109) expressed it, the mud will settle and answers will become clear.

Ifs and buts

We have arrived at a critical point. You are about to embark on the process of becoming aware of your values. You are on the verge of taking steps that will help you live according to your values. It is very likely that you will have to make crucial decisions. You are actually setting out on the route through your landscape of values. This is when the baggage in your backpack may start to make its presence felt and to bother you again. Here are some examples of typical ifs and buts. Do you recognize them?

But if I start to live like that I'll be fired. I'm much too busy. We estimate this to be one of the most common reservations. It is the spirit of the times. Everyone and everything around us is in doing mode, so we seem unable to permit ourselves to be in being mode. Consider the following:

⇒ Living with attention is not the same as being passive or lazy.
⇒ Sometimes your insecurity or anxiety is more in your head than in reality.
⇒ Explore and try. Start with one day in the week. Then continue from there.

- By doing things calmly and with attention, you can start to work more efficiently.
- It's about leading a meaningful and satisfying life. If your work conflicts too much with your values, perhaps it's time for a change?
- Who knows what kind of positive effect it will have on those around you!

The time's not right, I'm not ready yet. Maybe tomorrow, the day after, later.

This is so typical of experiential avoidance! Acknowledge your feelings. Name them and accept them, but don't let them take the helm! Remember, you can't be 'half ready'.

I don't know what my real values are.

This is a sneaky excuse. Of course you know.

- Really project yourself into it: how would you lead your life if you knew you'd be dead in a year's time?
- Try your coffin on for size: imagine your loved ones gathered around the grave and look them in the eye. What would you want them to say about you?
- Deep down inside, you do know what really matters to you.

Don't let your mind mess you around.

I can't do it; it'll just go wrong again.

OK, it's the 'I can't do it' scenario again, the 'disaster scenario'. I was expecting you. Welcome. Where have you been? I've listened to you carefully, but do you mind if I do my own thing now? Thank you.

If you think about it closely, you will notice that all of these ifs and buts are actually forms of experiential avoidance. They often point to a fear of the consequences that living according to your values will entail, so you can often boil them down in turn to whether or not you are ready to experience sadness, insecurity, anxiety, etc.

Whenever you find yourself confronted with ifs and buts, try to apply the following.

➡ Name and accept your doubts, insecurities, anxieties, etc.
➡ Don't be drawn into a debate, take the step you want to take.
➡ You can't haggle with your values. Half a life is no life.
➡ Identify your typifying thoughts. Call them by their name. Say 'thank you' to your mind.
➡ Always remember: this is only the first step. We are not asking you to turn your whole life upside down straight away.

Once you've discovered your values and know what choices go with them, once you've acknowledged and accepted the accompanying doubts, insecurities and anxieties, and are ready to carry them on board without letting them take the helm, you will have taken the biggest step, made the leap. Now you need to steer a straight course, to give your meaningful life a chance to really take root and grow into that magnificent, strong, distinctive tree.

Exercise: list of areas of life and values

This exercise (Hayes et al. 1999) helps you to gain an idea of values that matter to you in different areas of life and to choose where you want to begin the process of living according to your values. To help you, here is a list of examples of values.* You can of course add other values that are not on the list but are important to you.

* Based on the Rokeach Value Survey (Johnston 1995).

Action	Peace
Altruism	Pleasure
Capability	Power
Cheerfulness	Punctuality
Confidence	Responsibility
Courage	Security
Creativity	Self-assurance
Discipline	Self-development
Education	Sociability
Equilibrium	Sportsmanship
Faith	Success
Family	Sympathy
Freedom	Tolerance
Friendship	Truth
Harmony	Variety
Health	Wealth
Honesty	Work
Humour	....
Independence	....
Individuality	....
Joy	....
Justice	....
Love	....
Loyalty	....
Openness	....
Parenthood	....

Tip

If you find it difficult to choose on the basis of this list, it may also help to cut out 40 or more small cards from a sheet of paper. Write a value on each card. If you have extra values, write these down as well. Then make three piles: values that matter to you very much, values you consider reasonably important and values that are not particularly important to you. Then, from the first pile, choose three values that matter to you most.

The following table contains 11 areas of life. We want you to give each area a rating, in the second column, of between 1 and 10. If you rate it a 1, the area is completely unimportant to you; an area that scores a 10 is extremely important. You needn't prioritize, so you can give each area a 10 if you like.

In the third column, write down some values that matter to you in that area of life. In the fourth column, rate the extent to which you believe you are living according to your values at this moment. If you believe you are living fully in line with your values, enter a 10; if you believe you are completely failing in this respect, write down a 1.

Area of life	Extent to which this area matters to you	Values	Extent to which you are living according to your values in this area
Family			
Marriage/ intimate relationships			
Parenthood			
Friends/social life			

Area of life	Extent to which this area matters to you	Values	Extent to which you are living according to your values in this area
Work			
Education/ training			
Physical care			
Participation in groups or associations			
Belief/ Spirituality			
Leisure/ Relaxation			
Contributing to society (in addition to paid employment)			

Choosing an area of life

Now we ask you, as a first step, to choose an area of life where you want to live closer to your values. One option is to choose an area that scored highly in terms of importance (in the second column), but lower in terms of living according to your values (in the fourth column).

Exercise: discovering values

The following section contains some additional exercises that can help you to discover your values. Choose an exercise that appeals to you. You may discover that the values you have chosen are indeed the ones that matter most to you, or you may discover new values. Equally, you may discover that you'd rather work on a different area of life first.

Exercise 1

Start by answering the following question: what do I want out of life?

The intention now is that you keep asking yourself 'why', 'what' and 'for what purpose', until you come across a value. When you ask yourself questions, goals lead you automatically to values. The following example is based on Harris (2007):

What do I want out of life?
If I'm really honest, to be filthy rich.
Why do I want that?
Because then I can do whatever I want.
What would I do, for example?
Travel round the world.
What would that bring me?
I'd visit exotic countries and spend all day lounging on the beach.
What do I like about lying on the beach?
Relaxing! **(value)**
What could I do to get started right away?

We are not saying that getting rich shouldn't be a goal if that helps you live according to key values. However, constantly asking questions enables you to identify the values that belong with that goal. Why wait 10 years to apply those values (running the huge risk that you won't succeed in achieving that goal) if you can take the first step straight away? If you really want to laze on a beach in a far-away country, it makes sense to start saving. Don't hesitate to apply your key value right here, right now.

Another example:

What do I want out of life?
If I'm really honest, to be filthy rich.
Why do I want that?
Because then people will look up to me.
Why is that important to me?
Then they'll treat me better, at least I'll get some respect.
What would that bring me?
I'd be more at ease, I could be more myself **(value)**.
What could I start doing now in order to be myself?
I could ask myself who makes me feel at ease, and who doesn't.

That's a good idea. What else?
I'm only going to associate with people I can be myself with.

Give it a try: keep asking yourself these questions until you come across a value.

What do I want out of life?

....

....

....

....

....

....

....

....

Exercise 2

Look back over your life. Ask yourself the following questions:

➠ Can you remember times or periods when you felt inspired, when your heart opened up, when you felt moved? Why was that the case? Which values played a role?

➠ Which films, books or conversations really touched you?
Why was that the case? What chord did they touch in you?
What does that say about your values?

➠ Who have you admired, or do you admire now? Why is
that? What does that person stand for? Can you boil that
down to values that matter to you?

Your motto or watchword

This week you have been working with your values. Could you sum up and put into words what you have discovered so far? Is there a particular statement or image that could serve as your motto or watchword?

Write this motto down below.

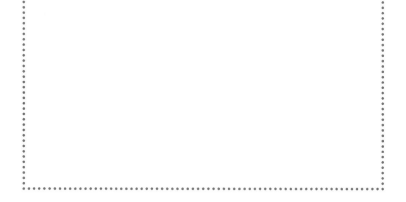

Mindfulness exercise: routine exercise with attention

All day long, we face a variety of tasks. Most of our actions are done on automatic pilot. Carrying out one or more day-to-day activities with attention can help you to develop your awareness and attentiveness. Everyday habits are experienced more consciously. This may help you to realize that certain actions and behaviours are ingrained patterns. In many cases, of course, this is not a problem (e.g. changing gear while driving, cleaning your teeth). But there are also some ingrained, automatic patterns that are not good for us. Overeating due to stress, for example. Nail biting, constantly butting heads with people, continually overstepping the mark or being led astray.

Choose one activity that you are going to do with attention for the following week. This can be an activity with a pattern that you might want to change in the long run. It can also be an everyday routine activity (such as cooking, putting out the rubbish, watering plants or taking a shower). In the latter case, the attentiveness is bound to spread to other activities as well.

If you choose an activity that you might want to change, remember that the exercise is primarily about becoming aware. What does the pattern look like? What do you notice from moment to moment? Try to observe this in a gentle manner. Try not to change the behaviour as you observe it. By developing attentiveness, this moment will come of itself.

Example: teeth cleaning

Be aware of each individual action. Walking to the washbasin, picking up the toothbrush, picking up the tube of toothpaste, opening the cap, putting toothpaste on the toothbrush, putting down the tube, bringing the toothbrush to your mouth, tasting and smelling the toothpaste, brushing carefully, spitting, rinsing out, putting away the toothbrush.

Example: nail biting

The first thing to say is that you probably don't become aware of nail biting until you're already doing it. Notice that. Observe what you are doing. What exactly *are* you doing, what do you perceive, what feelings or sensations do you have, etc. The more often you do this, the more you will notice what precedes the nail biting and what happens afterwards, which will allow you to discover patterns in this ingrained behaviour. Awareness may cause the behaviour to diminish. This happens because space is created between the pattern and yourself: space that gives you the option of breaking the habit.

Walking with attention

Walking (outdoors) is an ideal activity to do with attention. This exercise can be done slowly or at a normal pace. Anything from a minute to an hour is fine. Here are two variations, options for observing the movement of the feet:

⇒ Left, right, left, right. . .
⇒ Up, down, up, down. . .

3

Authenticity

The famous German philosopher Martin Heidegger wrote at length about ways of leading your life and being in the world.*

On the one hand, we are 'thrown' into an existing world. We live in a family, country and culture with particular norms, values and customs that we adopt without being aware of it. These are behaviours that many people in a particular environment have in common. For example, thriftiness and a strong work ethic are traits that the Dutch and the Scots are said to have in common. But language too will shape our shared experience and view of the world. You could sum this up as what is 'given': everything that is already there.

On the other hand, life also holds out a range of possibilities and we have the freedom to make personal choices and follow our own path. We can be aware of the meaning of our behaviour; we may feel that we have a particular role to play, that life has a purpose, one to which we can contribute. We find that the decisions we take make a difference. We feel a sense of responsibility.

According to Heidegger, a person's life is 'inauthentic' if he conforms to social norms unthinkingly and lets himself be guided by other people or the community. It is a life in which

* Based on Guignon (2002).

he becomes wrapped up in the everyday hustle and bustle without taking time for reflection. A person's life becomes authentic when he starts to consciously choose options that life offers. If he thinks about values (chosen life directions) and takes responsibility for them, clarity and energy are the result.

Authenticity implies an absence of egotism. It is about a greater awareness of being part of a history and a larger context, but we are also more aware of how we can make a contribution.

Week 8
Go for it!

Life is not a dress rehearsal.
Rose Tremain

Introduction

And now we come to the crunch. Are you ready to go for it? You have made all the preparations you need in order to live life in the moment (according to your values). You have been honest with yourself in confronting your tendency to live half a life on the basis of avoidance. You have realized that it didn't take you any closer to the life you want to lead. You have practised a number of important aids such as acceptance, readiness to experience what is there, mindfulness and cognitive defusion. You have started to realize that you are not the sum of your achievements, thoughts or possessions and that you are, above all, the ever-present ability to experience and be aware. And you have identified the values that, for you, are the vital ingredients of a worthwhile and authentic life: values that make life worth living for you and give you a purpose and direction in life. Now it is crunch time. This week, you will decide the first steps you want to take, and actually take them. '*Walk the talk*', you might say. Act according to your values. Deeds not words.

Sarah is a lawyer with two children. She worked hard to get through her studies; she didn't really enjoy the course and it took her a lot of effort. It was her parent's wish that she should go to university, as they had never had that opportunity themselves. She felt proud to work as a lawyer and did enjoy the respect it commanded.

However, she often feels gloomy and guilty. She thinks she should be enjoying her children more. She has nothing to complain about, after all. Her manager finds her lacking in motivation and they come to a clash. Sarah believes she's doing her best. It makes her furious to think her manager doesn't see it. When she finally ends up at the company doctor, who recommends a training course to help her find out what she actually wants, it comes as a relief. The shoe has been pinching for years as a matter of fact.

Sarah is aware that she is pushing herself to the limit. This is a familiar pattern for her. Looking at her reasons for going to university, she realizes that the impetus didn't come from herself. She'd much rather have chosen a creative profession and thinks her talents would have been much better served by a vocational course.

At the moment her family is the main priority. Because she is often down, she is short with the children. Sarah takes a number of radical decisions. She decides to cut her hours and enrols in a silversmithing course. The financial consequences are significant, but she finds she can still get by and money isn't actually that important to her. Some of her friends don't understand her decision, so one or two of them fall by the wayside.

Although the consequences are difficult at first, she also notices the benefits. Going to her course makes her feel cheerful and energized. And she is able to laugh at her children's antics again. In retrospect, she is pleased that she clashed with her manager. Otherwise, she wouldn't have made any of these changes.

Exercise: defining actions

Last week you thought about your main areas of your life and the values that matter to you most in those areas. You have 'coloured in' your landscape of living in the moment with actual values. The key is now to apply those values in practice: in other words, you actually have to enter that landscape. You also chose an area of life that you plan to work on first, and thought about the values that matter to you most in that area. What action or actions can you take in the short term in order to live more in line with your values in this area?

Action 1

Action 2

Action 3

Make sure these actions are concrete and feasible. By 'concrete', we mean they should be actual behaviours. For example, you may decide to pursue further development at work because learning is a value that matters to you and you are finding your work too routine at the moment. This intention becomes concrete when you have a meeting with your boss to announce it, or when you sign up for career counselling to find out what exactly it is you want, or when you embark on further training or a refresher course.

This example shows that it is sometimes necessary to break an action down into chunks. In the above example, a first step might be to have an exploratory meeting with your boss to see if he or she is prepared to work with you on this.

Exercise: defining ifs and buts

Before carrying out your actions, it is important to prepare for the ifs and buts that accompany them. It is not about conquering these ifs and buts at the outset. You are going to carry out your action while putting up with them. You are not going to let them tell you what to do.

What thoughts might try to stand in your way?

What emotions might crop up, both before and during your action?

You can prepare for these ifs and buts by practising cognitive defusion and mindfulness exercises (e.g. 'making space for what is there'). Are you prepared to actually experience the negative emotions (anxiety, doubt, insecurity) that accompany the action? Make sure your ifs and buts don't start to regain control of your life (see also the tour guide metaphor discussed below).

Exercise: carry out your actions – time to set off

The next step is to actually carry out a few of your actions. Here are some tips.

- ➟ Try giving yourself a reminder that will help you persevere with your action despite the best endeavours of your ifs and buts. For example, carry around with you a card on which you have written your motto or key value or an object that acts as a symbol for your motto.
- ➟ Don't put off your actions. Putting things off is often an attempt to 'do a deal' with living in the moment.
- ➟ Don't fixate on the outcome. It's all about the journey. It's about taking steps that fit in with your values. You can't know at this stage exactly where the path will lead you.
- ➟ Prepare yourself for ifs and buts from those around you: it is not just you who can put obstacles in your path. What objections or questions might stem from someone else? How can you respond to them? How can you show other people that you really mean it?

Mindfulness exercise: everything in one

In previous mindfulness exercises you focused your attention on one specific object, such as physical sensations, thoughts or the breath. In the following exercise you are not going to focus on anything in particular. A succession of experiences will come forward. When an experience comes to the fore, focus your attention on it for as long as it remains there.

- ⇒ Sit down in your usual position and set an alarm.
- ⇒ Focus your attention first on your breathing. Notice how the breath flows in and out of your body.
- ⇒ Now be aware of what is happening within you from moment to moment.
- ⇒ If there are thoughts, observe your thinking; if there are sounds, observe your hearing; if there are sensations, observe the sensations; if there are emotions, observe your emotions; and so on.
- ⇒ Open yourself up and be present with everything that comes to the fore from moment to moment.
- ⇒ You don't need to do anything, just be open-minded and present with everything that is there.
- ⇒ If nothing comes to the forefront for a while, focus your attention on the breath. As soon as another object presents itself, focus your attention on it.
- ⇒ This method may help you to experience something of the basis of 'being': a state in which you are not required to do anything but are simply an observer of what is taking place in the now.

Metaphor: the tour guide

Now imagine the following. This week you have actually set foot in your landscape of living in the moment. You have decided what direction you want to go in, with your values acting as a compass. In the distance you can see a hilltop or a tree that serves as a reference point. And now you have set off, ready to carry out your actions.

But you are not alone on your walk. A procession of ifs and buts is trailing in your wake. And the further you go, the more the party starts to clamour, and to tug and shout at you. One says you'll never make it, you'll get lost. A second tells you to turn right, although *you* know it should be left. The next predicts an attack or robbery. The fourth in line reminds you how safe and comfortable it is back at home. The fifth forecasts bad weather and warns you that you had better turn round.

Can you imagine yourself in this situation? What do you do? How, as a tour guide, are you going to handle your group of difficult tourists? Write your reactions down below.

Continue to page 154.

Dying without regrets

The philosopher Nietzsche had another question that may help you in actually carrying out your intended actions. Indeed, it is perhaps the most important question you can ask yourself at any moment: imagine you don't manage to live according to your values or to carry out your intended action; looking back in 5 years' time, would you have any regrets? Are you prepared to risk that?

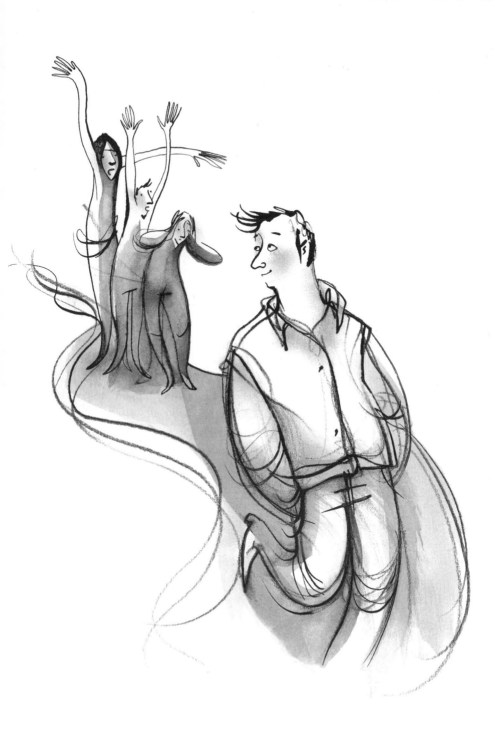

Isn't this the worst thing that can happen to a person, to be lying on their deathbed and having regrets about their life because they haven't lived to the full, haven't done what they knew in their heart they should have done?

There is only one time when you can prevent that, and it is now.

Metaphor: the tour guide (continued)

There are a number of options. You can enter into a debate with your ifs and buts. You can try to convince them that you know where you're going and have made thorough preparations. But what happens then? You stop walking; that in itself pleases the party. An endless discussion ensues, because the ifs and buts simply won't be persuaded. As time goes on you begin to tire and become discouraged; you start to doubt your mission. Perhaps it *is* better to turn right; it's true, there *are* dark clouds on the horizon. And you decide to turn back for now, so you can talk it all through and then start over again. Now the ifs and buts are really delighted. They cluster cheerfully around you, cracking jokes and patting you on the back until, all too soon, you find yourself back at your starting point.

Or, you can adopt the stance of a friendly but determined tour guide. You keep walking. You look each member of the party squarely in the eye. 'I have listened to you closely, thanks for your advice, but I am going on.' And you continue at a brisk pace. The ifs and buts grumble for a while but reluctantly follow in your footsteps.

Now return to page 152.

Week 9
Keep going for it

Patience is the mark of love.
I do not believe there is one skill in life that is more valuable.
As far as I know, patience is the best protection against all
sorts of emotional and physical problems.
Eknath Easwaran

Introduction

Before you picked up this book, you had probably arrived at a
station aboard the train of thought. You were en route to a
terminus called 'Living Happily Ever After', but saw this for the fairy
tale it is and started to have doubts about your destination. So you
got out and boarded a new train.

This train is heading for a worthwhile, meaningful life. There is
no final destination anymore. As soon as you've left the station,
you are where you are supposed to be. It's all about the journey.
Your baggage of loneliness, anxiety and insecurity is on board too.
You are sharing a compartment with Mr Gloomy and Mrs Doubtful.
There's a good chance that other travellers of a similar persuasion
will join you along the way. And you will often stop at stations
where another train of thought awaits. Mr Gloomy and Mrs
Doubtful will try to get you to change trains. 'We'll just stay here
and won't bother you anymore,' they say.

But the decision is yours, and we hope you will stay put.
Because you know what you have to do. You have set yourself a
task. So thank them kindly for their advice and let the journey
continue, as you sit back and watch the countryside pass by.

You have reached the end of this book. Now it is over to you again. We would like to finish by giving a few more tips and ideas that may help you on your journey, in living according to your values.

Develop your own philosophy of life*

A few years ago the Dutch tax authorities had a slogan: 'We can't make it any more fun, but we can make it easier'. We could say something similar about the art of living: 'We can't make life any more fun, but we can make it fuller'. There is suffering in the world. There is insecurity, inequality and injustice. We all experience loss. We are all put on this earth to die. No one has a lease on the ultimate truth. We can't control our lives. One man will be dealt a larger portion of distress than his neighbour. Those are the basic ingredients of life and we simply have to deal with them.

The essence of this book is the realization that you can live in the moment only if you are prepared to experience distress, loss, insecurity and inequality. If you are prepared to do that, life does not become more fun *per se*, but it does become more intense, more authentic, more meaningful. When you are ready to play with the cards you have been dealt, you become rooted in your personal situation in life (your lot) and that enables you to grow into a strong and distinctive tree. And if you share this vision you will also realize that it doesn't matter in the end whether you were born in a glittering palace or a humble cottage.

The vital question, therefore, is how we relate to the basic ingredients of life. We believe that everyone develops their own philosophy of life. There are countless possible philosophies and beliefs, but two basic schools of opinion can be distinguished: 'Life is meaningless' and 'Life has meaning'.

The first philosophy holds that life is senseless and arbitrary.

* Based on Schmid (2007).

You may be lucky, or you may be unlucky. It is a philosophy that can degenerate into cynicism and hopelessness: whatever we do, none of it matters. This attitude can therefore tend to fuel feelings of bitterness, despondency and injustice, and may lead to detachment.

The second philosophy holds that, ultimately, there is sense in everything. However meaningless and unfathomable life may sometimes appear, there is a point to our lives: what we do matters. This attitude tends to invite empathy, connection and commitment. It is important to realize that both philosophies are no more than assumptions. There is no ultimate truth. There is no ultimate evidence for one or the other. You may be personally convinced, you may have experiences that you believe to be incontrovertibly true, but someone else may have quite different experiences or interpretations.

The question is, which assumption about life do you apply, and does it help to make your life worth living? In Week 7 we asked you to think about the values that matter to you. What we were actually doing was inviting you to develop or formulate a personal philosophy of life. It may help to take this a stage further in the future.

Temper your expectations

One of the biggest challenges about the art of living is not to expect too much. Expectations soon lead to disappointment and stop you seeing what is happening to you in the now.

Paul recounted once, during a training course, how he used to draw up a detailed plan based on travel guides whenever he was about to go on a trip. His schedule would take in all of the highlights mentioned in the guides. But it was always a bit disappointing in the end: everything was less beautiful and spectacular than he'd expected, based on the descriptions. For a couple of years now, he has only made very general plans. He allows himself to be guided by encounters, by spontaneous detours, by whatever crops up. His trips have now become more satisfying and somehow more special.

This is a good metaphor for life itself. Which is not to say that you shouldn't make plans any more and shouldn't have any expectations. The art is to leave enough room in your life planning for surprises, sudden changes of perspective, new routes. Bear in mind that what you've planned may not happen. 'Life is what happens to you while you're busy making other plans,' as John Lennon put it. The art of living is a dance: sometimes you take the lead and sometimes you are guided by what happens to you.

3

Prepare yourself for the fact that a new attitude to life will have consequences

When you think more deeply about your values and then start to live according to them, it is important to bear in mind that this may have consequences. You may discover that you want a change of job. You may take a path that isn't understood by some of your friends or your partner. You may end up losing friends or seeing them less often. This can be viewed as a necessary loss. If you can be aware of this, it may be easier to deal with. It is entirely possible that people around you will try to stop you doing what is important to you; they will warn you off, or tell you you're mad or foolish. Never disregard well-intentioned advice. Listen well, measure it against your values. But be prepared to not necessarily follow it.

It can be useful, therefore, to seek out allies: people who understand the process you are going through and what you want, and who can support you.

Perseverance: second nature

Living according to your values takes a lot of time and space at the start. After all, you are no longer living on automatic pilot! You have to be in constant touch with 'being' mode. It also takes a lot of perseverance, a lot of commitment, at the outset. Your values need time to 'take root', to burrow deeper into the ground.

In the long run it will become second nature to you. Once you have put your philosophy of life more into practice in the wider world, you will become a better judge of whether or not something suits you. Your intuition will go from strength to strength. You will know more readily what you need to do, or what you need to shed. You will become more decisive. But it can help to realize that this takes time. The art of living includes having the patience of a tree.

In this final week you will learn how to use a checklist to cope with difficult times. And we will give some tips for broadening your experience of living in the moment so that it does indeed become second nature to you.

We wish you *bon voyage* for the rest of your journey!

'Living in the moment' in a nutshell

In essence, you have got to know three aspects of yourself, and you have gradually set to work with them.

The first aspect is your talent for struggling. This includes your battle with psychological pain, your attempts to conquer distress. It is your fight or flight behaviour, which may have been effective in surviving in the outside world but doesn't work in our inner world because it tends to increase distress rather than reduce it. It is the route to regrets and victimhood. It is the route of saying 'no' to life.

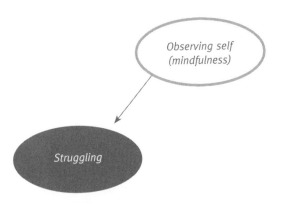

With the aid of mindfulness, you have started to notice your struggling. You do this using the second aspect: your ability to notice and observe. This is that part of yourself that is always there, no matter what you do. The observing self enables you to keep choosing between struggling or living according to your values.

3

Then you became aware of an alternative to a life centred around struggle: your talent for living according to your values (the third aspect). This is the ability to make choices based on your values and to act accordingly. It works because you experience more satisfaction, because you become more energetic and authentic. It encompasses both distress and pleasure. It is the route of readiness and heroism. It is the route of saying 'yes' to life.

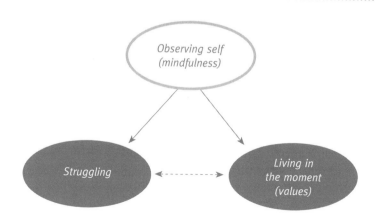

That, in essence, is the decision you face at every moment of the day. Either you struggle or you live in the moment according to your values. From now on, you will always be able to take time out to observe and be aware of which of these two options is at play in your life. This is also the basis of the following 'relapse checklist'.

Relapse checklist

Read the following through carefully, even if you are currently living in the moment. This will help you to retrieve the checklist quickly in future if you find you're no longer living (temporarily) in the moment.

The summary on the previous pages also provides guidelines for handling relapses. A relapse is to be expected: it's only human. As we said in the summary, there are always two options: either you live according to your values or you struggle. In the former case you are living to the full; in the latter, you are half-living or not living at all.

What do we mean by a relapse? It means that struggling, fighting your psychological distress, has become central to your life again. This may express itself as increased avoidance of experiences. Or as an increase in fatigue, anxiety, gloominess, insecurity or anger. Or a feeling that you are a victim of your circumstances, that things are conspiring against you. A relapse may also manifest as an inability to carry out your actions on the basis of your values, or an inability or unwillingness to make decisions.

In the following pages, we outline a number of tips and questions that you can run through as a checklist when you find yourself falling back into old patterns.

1   *Congratulate yourself*
First of all, it is important to realize that you have noticed your 'relapse', a feeling that something is not right any more, that you have stopped being satisfied with your life. This is necessary, because otherwise you wouldn't be referring to this checklist. In realizing this you have already taken the most important step, because now you can do something about it again. If you're struggling without being aware of it, you can't change anything! Equally, this is a good reason for the second point on this checklist.

2   *Ask your partner or someone you trust to warn you*
Often, those who are close to you will realize you're having a relapse before you do. You may have told them about this book and the process you're going through. Ask them to alert you if they notice any specific behaviour that accompanies struggling in your case (avoidance, smoking, alcohol, etc.).

3   *Are you judging yourself?*
Try to stay kind to yourself. Everyone will have times when they try to lead half a life again, or get caught up in fighting their distress. That's only human. If you have been struggling for years, you won't get it out of your system quickly. It is bound to raise its head from time to time.

4   *Are you fighting clean pain in your life?*
Is there a particular emotion in your life? Sadness, disappointment, insecurity, anxiety, gloominess? You may have to go back in time a bit (a day, a week, a month) to get to the clean pain. Is there a particular time when that emotion emerged? What is it connected to? Is it possible that you are fighting that emotion, that it is the cause of your struggling? Can you accept this clean pain again? It may help to do the mindfulness exercise 'making space and allowing what is there'.

5   *Have you been living in 'doing mode' a lot?*
Sometimes, a relapse may occur because you've been really busy for a while and haven't taken enough time for mindfulness. You've allowed everyday life to swallow you up and haven't taken time out to experience what you want and think. At times like these, struggling can easily worm its way back into your life because you tend to see any negative thought or emotion as a disruption of your busy life, and you can do without that. The solution is obvious. Try in the short term to find some quiet time for mindfulness and contact with your observing self. If you can't manage that straight away, try at least to devote your full attention to what you are doing.

6   *Can you change anything about your circumstances?*
Think back to the saying by Teresa of Avila on page 77. You may be troubled by circumstances that you can change. Is that the case? If so, take action to change the things you can influence. If not, you will have to seek a solution in acceptance of the resulting emotions.

7   *Is your ego playing up?*
It is possible that you feel a strong need for recognition? Do you find yourself judging and comparing? We live in a society that is focused on performance and status, so it's not unusual

to be tempted to link our self-worth to achievements or possessions. It can help to be aware of this, and to take time to make contact with your observing self. Perhaps reintroduce a slower pace and a little more silence into your life. Practise 'staying small' again (see page 120).

8   *Have certain ifs or buts gained the upper hand?*
Have certain convictions or doubts taken hold in your mind? Have you boarded another train of thought? Write down your thoughts and see if you can apply cognitive defusion. It may help to do the mindfulness exercise 'observing your thinking'. Try again to see your thoughts as a waterfall; you can stand underneath it, but another option is to stand behind it.

3

9   *Is there opposition from those around you?*
Are there people who are trying to sabotage you or to tempt you into leading half a life, or who don't understand the routes you are taking through your landscape of living in the moment? Be firm and state your boundaries. They will have to accept you as you are. And if they don't, you may have to distance yourself from them or break contact with them (for a while).

10   *Stay active, expand your experience of living in the moment*
The main way to prevent a relapse is to keep going forward. Continue to live with attention. Meditate regularly. Strike out on new routes in the landscape of your values. Try to be like the 'guest house' (see page 80) every day. (See also below: What next?)

Whatever you notice, try to stay kind to yourself. There will still be a thousand times when you find yourself playing tug of war, debating with your ifs and buts, trying to inflate your ego, trying to lead half a life. But you will also have a thousand opportunities to live in the moment.

What next?

If you have spent years trying to lead half a life, a life full of avoidance, this will have left a deep impression. Over the past few weeks you have begun to carve out a new track in preparation for a new route. But the new track is not yet as deep as the old one. Especially at the start, it is easy to fall back into old tracks. In a sense, they are safe and familiar! This is why it is vital to actively maintain your new way of life as you go forward. It will help you to keep going on the new track until a time comes when you suddenly find it has become familiar to you.

We would like to end with a number of tips on where to go from here with what you have learnt in this book:

- Keep doing meditation exercises regularly. Or try enrolling for yoga or tai chi classes, which are also useful aids to help you to continue living with attention.
- Keep reading about living in the moment. Here are some examples of books that we sometimes refer to ourselves. Reading will help to keep you on the track of living in the moment.

    > Steven Hayes: *Get Out of your Head and into your Life* (2005)
    > Eckhart Tolle: *Practising the Power of Now* (2005)
    > Jeffrey Brantley: *Calming your Anxious Mind* (2007)

- Try to set to work looking at other areas of life, and to make choices based on your values, if you're not yet doing that satisfactorily in those areas. This will help you to add extra routes to your landscape of living in the moment.
- Seek out other people who are keen to live in the moment. You can help to keep each other on the right track. Make sure you spend enough time with them.

➠ Keep creating moments of silence in your life. This helps you to make contact with 'being mode' and your observing self. These are times when the 'mud can settle' and clarity and perspicacity can develop.

3

Glossary

Acceptance The readiness to experience pain, based on the awareness that distress is an inextricable part of living. Acceptance is not about throwing in the towel, not at all. It is about connecting with the situation as it is now. It is about situations you have no control over. You stop wasting energy on struggling and, at the same time, you take steps towards a more meaningful life. You focus your energies on the things you *can* change.

Automatic pilot Acting and thinking without conscious awareness. Many of our actions are automatic, such as changing gear while driving. This is useful because we no longer need to be aware of each individual action. But ingrained patterns of behaviour and thought can be harmful, in which case it makes sense to become aware of them. Only through awareness is change possible.

Cognitive defusion The thinker is able to view his thoughts from a distance and no longer identifies with them. He is aware that thoughts are merely events in the mind and no longer responds to them. Space has been created between the thinker and the thought. Thoughts are seen as parcels on a conveyor belt. In cognitive defusion, you stand beside the conveyor belt and watch the thoughts as they pass by. In cognitive fusion, you are constantly delving into the packages and lose sight of the bigger picture.

Commitment The degree to which you make decisions based on your values, and the degree to which you actually put your values into practice in the world through your behaviour. In other words, standing up for what you really want.

Coping   Behaviour focused on handling a problematic situation. There are a number of different coping styles, such as actively tackling the problem and seeking support. The more styles you have at your disposal, the better you are able to deal with problematic situations.

Doing mode/being mode   Doing mode is an active, driven state. In doing mode, you are constantly focused on a discrepancy between the current and the intended situation. You are obsessed with changing things, and try to achieve that. Often, you are preoccupied with the past and the future and are not living in the now. In being mode, you are able to allow what is there. Thoughts and feelings do not automatically trigger patterns of behaviour that are geared towards change. There is a greater ability to handle difficult situations. This mode is about balance. By spending more time in being mode, you can start to apply doing mode when it is really important and useful.

Experiential avoidance   Avoiding negative experiences. Shunning emotions such as anxiety, sadness, anger and pain. There are three forms of avoidance: relief (e.g. alcohol, food), prevention (e.g. avoiding difficult situations) and distraction (e.g. watching television, burying ourselves in work). Avoidance works in the short term but in the long term leads to more problems. Then, there is not only the negative experience but also 'dirty pain' as a result of the avoidance behaviour.

Mindfulness   Observing what presents itself from moment to moment, with open attention and without judging.

Observing self   The ability to observe events happening to oneself. The observing self has the ability to notice thoughts, emotions, behaviour, physical sensations and sensory stimuli (e.g. from the senses of hearing, touch and sight). When you are in touch with the observing self, you are aware that you are more than the sum of your thoughts, emotions, behaviour, etc. You can also see that the observing self is always there, and always was. The form you are living in (childhood to adulthood, the roles you play) differs, but the observing self is always the same. It can be likened to a sky full of clouds. The clouds change, but the sky stays itself.

Psychological flexibility   You are said to be psychologically flexible if you can apply the six components of ACT: if you accept psychological pain, manage not to identify with the content of your thoughts, live with attention, know that you are awareness first and foremost, know what your values are and live according to them. If you find yourself in a difficult situation in life and are psychologically flexible, you will notice that the situation influences you but doesn't throw you completely off your stride. You can continue to act effectively.

Values   Values are chosen life directions. They are not a goal with a final destination, but rather a standard you aim for. Values can change over time. If you are living according to your values, you will notice a feeling of lightness or relief. But if you are not, you may experience a feeling of heaviness or pressure. Something is not right, your heart isn't open.

Bibliography

Bommerez, J. (2007) *Minder Moeten, Meer Flow; Ontdek Opnieuw de Magie uit je Kinderjaren*. Eemnes, the Netherlands: Uitgeverij Nieuwe Dimensies.

Brantley, J. (2007) *Calming your Anxious Mind*, 2nd edn. Oakland, CA: New Harbinger Publications.

Coleman Barks (trans.) (2004) *The Essential Rumi*, new expanded edn. New York: Harper Collins.

Guignon, C. (2002) Hermeneutics, authenticity, and the aims of positive psychology, *Journal of Theoretical and Philosophical Psychology*, 22: 83–102.

Harris, R. (2007) *The Happiness Trap, Stop Struggling, Start Living*. Wollombi, Australia: Exisle Publishing.

Hayes, S. (2005) *Get Out of your Mind and into your Life*. Oakland, CA: New Harbinger Publications.

Hayes, S., Strosahl, K., Wilson, K. (1999) *Acceptance and Commitment Therapy: An Experiential Approach to Behaviour Change*. New York: Guilford Press.

Johnston, C.S. (1995) The Rokeach Value Survey: Underlying structure and multidimensional scaling, *Journal of Psychology*, 129 (5): 583–597.

Kabat-Zinn, J. (2001) *Full Catastrophe Living: How to Cope with Stress, Pain and Illness using Mindfulness Meditation*. New York: Random House Publishing Group.

Nietzsche, F. (1874) *The Gay Science* (trans. by W. Kaufmann). New York: Vintage.

Schmid, W. (2007) *Het volle Leven; 100 Fragmenten over Geluk*. Amsterdam: Ambo.

Segal, Z.V., Williams, J.M.G. and Teasdale, J.D. (2002) *Mindfulness-Based Cognitive Therapy for Depression: A New Approach to Preventing Relapse.* New York: Guilford Press.

Tolle, E. (2005) *Practising the Power of Now.* London: Hodder & Stoughton.

Tolle, E. (2009) *A New Earth.* London: Penguin.

Verduin, P. (1998) *De Vraag naar het Lichaam; Filosofie van Lichamelijkheid in de Gezondheidszorg.* Maarssen, the Netherlands: De Tijdstroom/Elsevier.